Guide Before You Start Exercising

First and foremost:

- You should be in good physical condition and be able to particip   ▁▁.
- Discuss with your doctor that you are planning to start this func▁   ..▁▁ rehabilitation programme. Follow their advice.
- Inform your next of kin that you are planning to start this programme.
- If you live with someone else, then let them know you are going to do some exercise. You could ask them to join you, or you could invite a friend. It is more fun if done with at least one other person; you can encourage and look after each other if needed.
- Have a phone very close by (ideally in your pocket) or any method of contact close to hand, especially if you are doing it alone. This is just so that you have options if you need some help at any time.

Where should I do the exercise?

- We recommend making sure that you choose a room with no obstructions on the floor. Make sure there are not any rugs that you could trip over! If you have a pet in the house, you might feel more comfortable if they are in another room so that you do not trip over them.

What should I wear?

- Make sure that you are dressed in comfortable clothes - nothing tight or restricting. Ensure that your trouser legs are hoisted up away from the floor so that you do not trip on the bottom. We recommend wearing trainers or shoes you feel comfortable in that fit well.

What should I eat beforehand?

- Eat about 1-2 hours before you start so that there is time for your food to digest, but not so long that you start to get hungry. It is good to keep some water and a small snack (for example, a banana) close to hand during the exercise workout.

What do I need to exercise?

- The exercises are designed to be done in a standard living room at home with minimal equipment. The only equipment you need are some chairs/table, ankle weights (1/2 or 1 kg on each leg) and exercise/resistance bands about 2 meters long (lighter and easy bands to start with). The ankle weights and exercise/resistance bands are available in most sports stores or online.

What about afterwards?

- It is normal to feel quite tired after the exercises - you have been moving your body and getting your heart pumping after all! Take it easy. Make sure to rest. It is vital to give your body time to recover before the next exercise.

Always listen to your body - you know yourself best, so trust your instincts! We are so glad to have you with us and we truly hope you enjoy the exercise guide.

Testimonials

"For many years I have had a bad back through wear, hard work, and sport. An MRI scan suggested that I needed a steroid injection. With 10 weeks to wait for my injection appointment, I started these classes... 8 weeks later I was pain free - walking miles and gardening all day... so I cancelled the appointment for the injection."

Female, 83

"I was diagnosed with a prolapsed disc. I attended the exercise classes and carried out the routine as instructed. I felt immediate benefits and I have been free of pain since."

Male, 81

"After attending the exercise classes I can only recommend that if you are suffering from pain or lack of mobility, you give them a try. These gentle exercises made such a difference to my life. I don't take medication and my quality of life has improved."

Female, 72

"Having suffered with a bad back for many years and previously using painkillers to relieve it, I was amazed that after regularly going to the exercise classes, my pain was relieved, and my back felt much stronger."

Male, 69

"Before attending the Free From Pain exercise classes, I had a painful left knee and mobility problems from near falls. But after attending the classes for about a year, my mobility improved tremendously. I can now go out for walks without pain and my near falls have stopped due to my strengthened thigh muscles."

Female, 78

"I attended these exercise classes following surgery for replacement of a broken hip. I have no doubt that the classes vastly helped in my recovery."

Male, 84

"I can now stand up without any assistance which I couldn't do before [the classes] and haven't fallen since. After starting the exercises my balance is much better. I found the exercises very helpful and enjoyable."

Female, 75

To all my patients who have taught me so much and have been the real encouragement to write this book and create the *Free From Pain* functional rehabilitation programme

To all my friends who supported me whilst I was putting this book together

To my friend and research assistant, Mr Jonathan Sims, whose help made this book possible

and

To Susan, Talita and Jemima for your constant inspiration, support and love

Free From Pain Exercise Book

Dr George Ampat
Consultant Orthopaedic Surgeon

Dr George Ampat FRCS works as a Consultant Orthopaedic Surgeon in the UK. After 30 years of surgical practice, he has taken a conscious decision not to operate. Dr. Ampat now aims to help patients with musculoskeletal pain with lifestyle changes, exercises, and diet rather than resorting to surgery.

DISCLAIMER – PLEASE READ THIS PRIOR TO USING THIS BOOK
Please note that the content of this book is for information only and is not a substitute for professional medical advice, diagnosis or treatment. It is strongly recommended that you consult with your doctor before beginning the *Free From Pain* or any exercise program. Do not start *Free From Pain* or any exercise program if your Doctor or other qualified health provider advises against it. You should be in good physical condition and should be able to participate in the exercise. You should understand that when participating in any exercise or exercise program, there is the possibility of physical injury. In addition, if you experience faintness, dizziness, pain or shortness of breath at any time while exercising, you should stop immediately and seek urgent medical advice. If you engage in this exercise or exercise program, you agree that you do so at your own risk and are voluntarily participating in these activities. To perform this exercise or exercise program in a safe way, you must make sure that the area you use is safe, flat, is clear of any obstacles, including edges of loose carpets and spacious enough for the type of activity.

Talita Cumi Ltd
681, Liverpool Road, Southport PR8 3NS
www.ampat.co.uk   www.freefrompain.org.uk

Printed in the United Kingdon

Ampat, George
Free From Pain, Exercise Book
ISBN 978-0-9956769-4-7

Table of Contents

Introduction

As a Consultant Orthopaedic Surgeon, I trained to operate on patients with arthritis, fractures, disc prolapses and other musculoskeletal issues. Surgery is essential in many situations but may not be needed in others. Over the course of my career, I noticed an increased dependence on surgery when the benefit did not meet the patient's expectations. In addition, surgery could cause complications. Having surgery is an irreversible decision. Hence, alternative options need to be considered before deciding to have a surgical procedure. There are many other less-invasive, risk-free interventions that can have similar or better outcomes than surgery. After practising surgical intervention for 25 years, I decided to give up surgery and explore how to help patients without surgical intervention. In order to help patients pursue a healthy life and avoid or even delay surgery, I became invested in providing alternative treatments, which do not involve going under the knife. One factor which is renowned for having a positive impact on health, musculoskeletal pain and life expectancy is exercise. During my career, I have seen first-hand how exercise can have huge benefits on patients' pain and general health. This is supported in the testimonials provided by patients of mine. I have therefore created the following exercise book to provide a set of exercises for each body part and guidance on how to complete them. This book is mainly aimed at seniors or adults who are over the age of 50. It can be used by others but is more focused on the over 50s who have pain in the bones and joints or generalised aches and pains.

The different exercise programmes

The *Free From Pain* functional rehabilitation programme is a fusion of three established exercise programmes. The Otago exercise programme for improving balance and increasing the strength of the leg muscles, the motor control exercises to help with lower back pain and the isometric and strengthening exercises to help with neck and shoulder pain. To begin with, follow the programme for 12 weeks. Each week read one reason and one metaphor and do the exercises on three or five days each week. Once you have been through the 12-week programme and you like it, then just repeat the exercises as a normal routine either three or five times each week. You ideally should not stop exercising. It is like brushing one's teeth. You should do it routinely.

This book has four parts. In the first part, I will explore the 12 reasons and 12 metaphors to inspire and encourage you to exercise. In the second and the third parts, I will provide exercises for the neck and lower back. The fourth and final part consists of exercises from the Otago exercise programme. This programme originated in Otago, New Zealand and was originally designed to reduce falls and improve balance in seniors. As a secondary consequence, the exercises also built muscular strength and helped to reduce pain.

I have referenced each section with peer-reviewed medical articles. Many of them are freely available on the Internet. Feel free to use the links to gather more information.

How often do I do the exercises?

There are two possible routines in which you can do the exercises. The first possible routine would be to do the entirety of the exercises three times a week. In this routine, you will be exercising three days a week and resting for four days. The alternative and the preferred routine would be to do the neck and back exercises twice a week and the Otago exercises three times a week. In this routine, you will be exercising five days a week and resting for two days.

The ideal five-day plan would be as follows:
Monday – Otago exercises
Tuesday – Neck and Back exercises
Wednesday – Otago exercises
Thursday – Rest day
Friday – Neck and Back exercises
Saturday – Otago exercises
Sunday – Rest day

You can choose either the five-day plan or the three-day plan. It is important that you choose the plan that suits you.

Can I push myself?

Whilst it is important that you are enthusiastic and need the determination to do the exercises regularly, you should not do "too much too soon". You should only do what you can. Doing too much may cause injury and further pain, which will discourage you from continuing to exercise. This is no good for anyone, as you will not reap the benefits that come with completing the programme.

The traffic light system

Think of a traffic light system. When the light is on green, you can go through the lights. If the light is on amber, you should be preparing to stop. If the light is on red, you should stop entirely. This is the same with the discomfort you may experience whilst exercising. If you are not experiencing pain or only mild discomfort, then you may continue to exercise as the light is on green. However, as soon as the discomfort increases and starts to become painful, you should prepare to stop as the light has changed to amber. It is better to stop completely at this stage than to carry on until the discomfort is severe and the light is on red. Doing so will prevent the pain cycle from kicking in. This will also allow you to carry on with the exercise programme when you have rested and are able to do so.

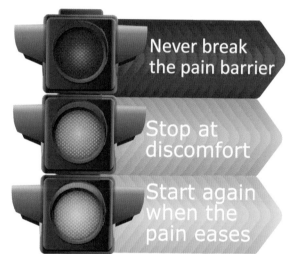

Never break the pain barrier

Stop at discomfort

Start again when the pain eases

The traffic light system should be used when you exercise. If you notice discomfort during exercise, stop and wait for a few minutes. Just like how the traffic light changes to green, the pain will decrease and you can start exercising again. Please do not go through the red light or break the pain barrier.

You can do it

I have been using this programme or parts of it for my patients over the last few years. With the right encouragement, a lot of them have been successful. Though the programme is good, the success rate has been only due to the positive outlook of my patients. The fact that you are reading this shows your keenness to improve your situation and get better. Please remain optimistic. I have every faith in you. I have seen a great many patients who felt their situation was impossible. They have managed to improve their health and mobility. With time and with slow and steady progress, we will win; I know you can do this. Please remain positive and hopeful. That is all I desire of you.

What if I fail or miss a few weeks?

It does not matter. The inability to adhere to an exercise schedule is very common. If you have missed a few days, a few weeks or even a few months, it does not matter. Just start the programme where you left it. If you have missed a whole year or even a few years, you can restart the entire programme once again. We all want to get better, but life gets in the way, and there are interruptions. This is completely understandable. Just restart when and where you can.

Additional information

You can view how to do the exercises on YouTube. Our channel is www.youtube.com/c/GeorgeAmpat The *Free From Pain* playlist in this channel provides all the videos of the exercises.

If you want to know more about lifestyle principles and how they can help you to decrease pain and live healthily, you may want to also read the book *"Free From Pain – Health Guide"*.

This is available separately at Amazon or on www.freefrompain.org.uk.

Online classes

You can also join the online exercise programme if you would find that suitable. Details on how to join the online classes are available at www.freefrompain.org.uk.

Combining the knowledge gained from the information book with the fitness and muscular strength acquired from following the exercise regime will give you many health benefits. For example, we hope to see reduced pain and improved mobility. As a result of these improvements, you will be more active and happier in your later life, whilst also extending your life expectancy.

I am very excited to invite you on this journey to live a life Free From Pain.

Dr George Ampat

The Size of the Problem

In the UK, the ageing population is growing as a result of increasing life expectancy. In 1920, life expectancy for men was 55 and for women was 59. In 2019, only 100 years later, men can now expect to live till 79.9 years, while women's life expectancy has increased to 83.6 years [1]. These improvements in life expectancy have been so remarkable that humans have now achieved biblical prophecy. Psalm 90:10 (New International Version) states, "Our days may come to seventy years, or eighty if our strength endures".

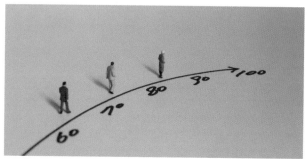

Life expectancy has increased over the last century

In line with increasing life expectancy, the number of older adults aged 65 and over who need care is also rising. In 2015, 2.2 million people over the age of 65 required care in England and Wales. This figure will increase by 25% to 2.8 million by 2025 [2].

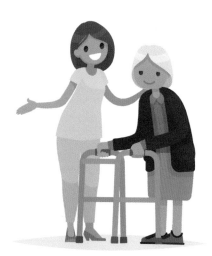

With these increases, more money and attention are needed to fund and manage the care and treatment of the elderly. It is therefore important that we endeavour to make later life as carefree as possible. Not only will this benefit individuals, but also society as a whole, through reducing the spending on later-life care and the strain on health services.

The goal is to lead healthier and fruitful lives even when we age.

References

1. Raleigh V. What is happening to life expectancy in the UK? The Kings Fund. 26 June 2020.
2. Guzman-Castillo M, Ahmadi-Abhari S, Bandosz P, et al. Forecasted trends in disability and life expectancy in England and Wales up to 2025: a modelling study. Lancet Public Health. 2017;2(7).

Reason 1 – Exercise Helps Us to Age Healthily Rather Than Gracefully

With the phrase "ageing gracefully", images of relaxing and happy seniors spring to mind. However, ageing gracefully seems to imply that one is accepting the limitations that come with age.

On the contrary, ageing healthily seems to imply just the opposite. Ageing healthily suggests that our later years are active and free from disability, where we can have independence and remain engaged in our community.

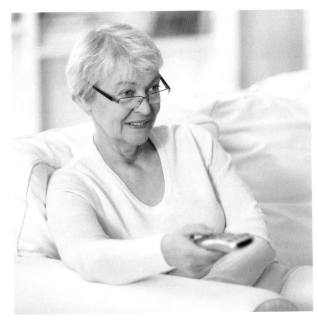

Ageing gracefully - increased sedentary time by watching TV

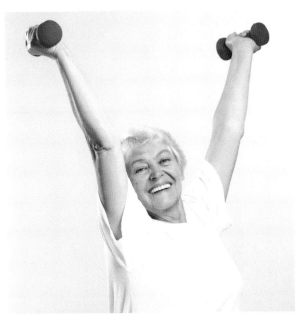

Ageing healthily – associated with increased activity

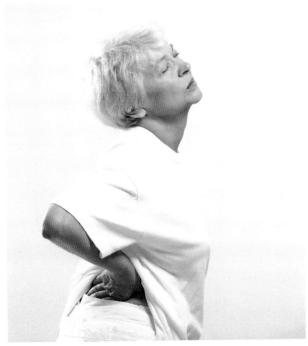

Ageing gracefully – less activity with increasing aches and pains

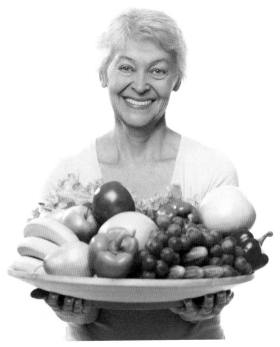

Ageing healthily – associated with consuming plant-based foods

In other words, later life should be a period of sustained health and vitality rather than a time of ill health and dependency.

The goal should be to age healthily with vitality and not to age gracefully with inactivity. One of the recognised solutions to address the adverse effects of ageing is exercise. Muscular activity and exercise are known to preserve brain function and memory [1].

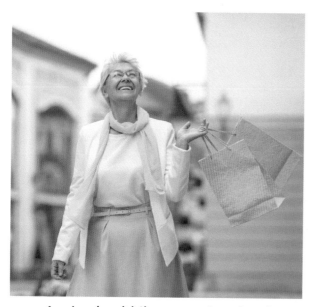

Ageing healthily – associated with increased productivity and life satisfaction

This is not dependent on the type of exercise. All modes of exercise, including aerobic exercise, dance and martial arts have been shown to improve memory function in all age groups [1]. Even moderately strenuous housework like gardening and cleaning is beneficial. Exercise drives neural activity in the brain and enhances the brain's ability to function [1]. To keep our brains functioning as we age, it seems that exercise is crucial.

References

1. Dause TJ, Kirby ED. Aging gracefully: social engagement joins exercise and enrichment as a key lifestyle factor in resistance to age-related cognitive decline. Neural Regen Res. 2019;14(1):39-42.

Metaphor 1 – How Can I Prevent Injuring My Back?

What is the story?

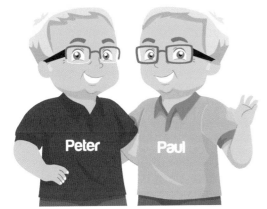

Peter and Paul are identical twins with the same genetic makeup. At the age of 40, they still look alike but have had very different jobs.

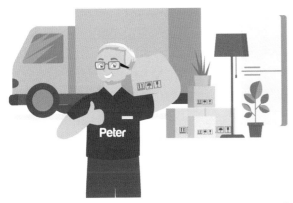

Peter worked in a removals company and lifted a total of four tonnes every day, moving boxes from the house to the van and from the van to the house.

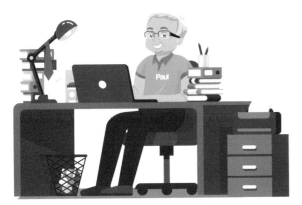

Paul, however, worked in an office and had a largely sedentary lifestyle.

One weekend they both decided to do some gardening and, as part of this, they needed to move some potted plants, which weighed around 20kgs.

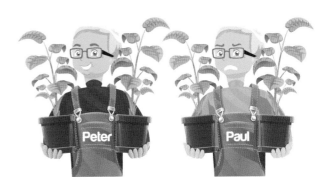

Peter had no problem when lifting the pots, but Paul struggled and injured his back. In the end, Paul blamed the lifting as the cause of his back pain.

So, what went wrong?

It may be easy to say the act of lifting caused Paul to hurt his back. However, if lifting were the cause of the back pain, then Peter, who lifts much more than Paul, would have had more chances of a back injury. It is possible that Paul was not fit to lift and that is why he hurt his back.

How can we relate this story to our health?

Our backs need to be strong to be supported and protected from injury.

To strengthen our backs, we must exercise regularly and only then should we attempt to lift heavy items. Once we have trained our backs, it will be much easier and safer to move heavy objects.

Moral of the story

Be fit and only then lift.

Reason 2 – Exercise Reduces Pain and Functions as a Pain Killer

Pain can result from injury or inflammation. When there is pain in a certain place, the basic instinct is to not move that body part through fear of making the pain worse. However, in the long term, avoiding movement or exercise does more harm than good. The lack of movement will cause the muscles surrounding the body part to become weaker. The weakness will reduce the support the muscles are able to provide to the joints, therefore increasing the pain and risk of further injury. A vicious cycle sets in and needs to be broken.

The difficulty is that exercise can both cause pain and relieve pain. However, it is known that long bursts of unaccustomed activity are likely to increase pain, whereas regular and short periods of accustomed activity are less likely to have this adverse effect. In fact, prescribed exercise is an effective treatment for most painful conditions [1]. The key is to slowly and incrementally increase the duration and intensity of exercise. Finding the right balance is essential.

How is pain transmitted within the body?

Imagine a needle prick to the finger. Sensory organs in the fingertip recognise the injury and send the signal through a nerve cell called a neuron. It takes three neurons and two junctions for the pain signal to travel from the finger and finally reach the brain. A neuron is a long structure. The first of the three neurons involved in the transfer of the signal starts at the skin and runs through the body, stopping just inside the spinal cord. It then transmits the signal to a second neuron via a junction. The signal is transmitted through the junction using chemicals called neurotransmitters. Once the second neuron has received the signal, it then sends it to the base of the brain, where there is a second junction. After passing this second junction, the signal then goes through a third neuron from the base of the brain to the area of the brain which detects pain. It is only then that the brain recognises that a needle has pricked the finger, causing the painful sensation. It takes a long time to describe this process, but the transfer of the signal is extremely quick in real-time.

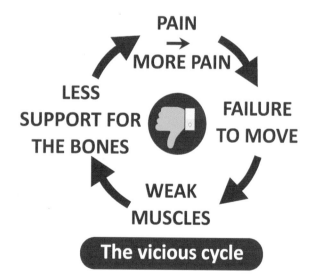

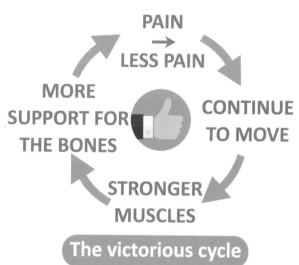

The vicous cycle needs to be converted into a victorious cycle

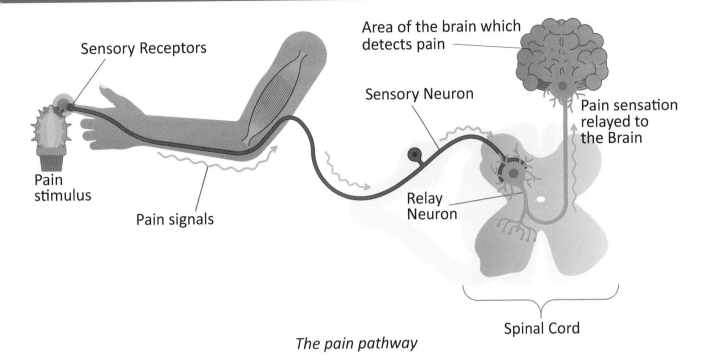

The pain pathway

Along this path, especially at the junctions, the signal can be enhanced (amplified) or suppressed (dampened). This modulation of the signal is akin to how a drum can be made to sound louder or quieter. When a drum is struck, a sound is heard. Tightening the drumhead will increase the sound, whilst loosening the drumhead will dampen it. Similarly, structures within the brain can enhance or dampen the pain signal. In cases of chronic pain, the brain enhances the pain signal. This causes even mild touch to be felt as severe pain. However, the good news is that regular exercise can dampen the pain signal, reducing the severity of pain sensation.

Exercise functions as a painkiller
In addition, exercise also acts as a painkiller and mood elevator [2]. This may be occurring through what is known as the endocannabinoid system [3]. It is well known that cannabis is a psychoactive drug that contains the active chemical cannabinoid.

Interestingly, recent research has found that the body itself can produce substances that are similar to the cannabinoid present in marijuana. The substance produced by the body is called endogenous cannabinoid, levels of which increase with exercise [3]. This is how physical activity produces an elevation in mood or a "high". This "high" might be the reason why some individuals get addicted to exercise. Cannabinoids, in addition to giving the "high", also reduce the pain sensation.

However, there is no recommendation for the consumption of cannabis. Cannabis consumption is harmful to health. We are only discussing here endocannabinoids produced naturally in the body.

As stated earlier, the intensity and duration of exercise must only be increased slowly over a period of time. "Too much too soon" would be a "boom and bust". With consistent, gradual increases, the "vicious cycle" can be converted into a "victorious cycle".

Too much too fast, will be a boom and bust,
But if the muscles sit and rest, the joints will only rust,
So, in your diary, find a space,
To exercise in any place,
A regular, consistent, and increasing pace
Will help you succeed and win the race.

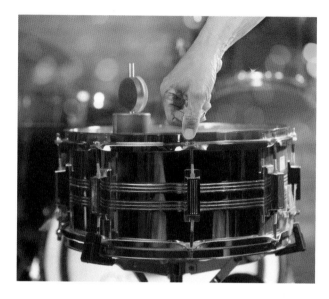

Tightening a drumhead increases the volume of the sound. Loosening the drumhead will decrease the volume of the sound.

References

1. Sluka KA, Frey-Law L, Hoeger Bement M. Exercise-induced pain and analgesia? Underlying mechanisms and clinical translation. Pain. 2018;159 Suppl 1(Suppl 1):S91-S97.
2. Naugle KM, Fillingim RB, Riley JL 3rd. A meta-analytic review of the hypoalgesic effects of exercise. J Pain. 2012;13(12):1139-1150.
3. Watkins BA. Endocannabinoids, exercise, pain, and a path to health with aging. Mol Aspects Med. 2018;64:68-78.

Metaphor 2 – My Back Feels Weak, Can I Make It Strong Very Quickly?

What is the story?

Patricia was late for work. She was worried about missing her meeting, so she drove above the speed limit down the motorway. She was caught by the police and fined for speeding. She ended up missing her whole meeting and had to pay the speeding fine.

So, what went wrong?

Patricia believed that the quickest solution to the problem would be to speed down the motorway. If she had followed the rules of the road and remained within the speed limits, she might have reached her workplace in adequate time and without the consequence of a speeding fine.

How can we relate this story to our health?

When patients first injure their back or any other body part, some are incredibly keen to get up and be active straight away. Activity is essential, but too much too soon is not good.

We need to pace ourselves to prevent further injury. It is essential to exercise in a controlled manner and gradually increase the intensity as our tolerance levels rise.

Moral of the story

After injury, too much too fast will be a "boom and bust".

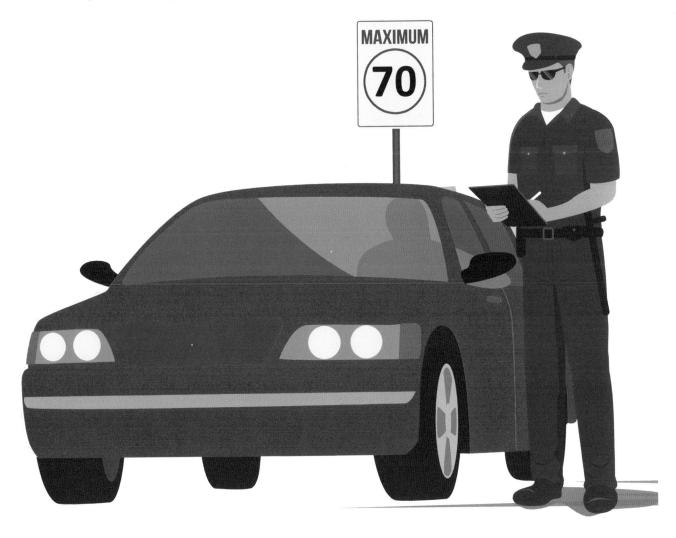

Reason 3 – Exercise Improves Bone Health and Reduces Hip Fractures

Osteoporosis

Ageing causes huge transitions and changes to the human body. One of these changes is that our bones become thin and fragile. In the early stages, when the bones become thinner, the condition is called osteopaenia. When the thinning becomes more severe, the condition is referred to as osteoporosis.

How does this happen?

Bone in the body is in a constant state of turnover. The body removes the old bone and replaces it with new bone. With ageing, the amount of old bone removed exceeds the amount of new bone that is formed. This is why the bones become thin, or "osteoporotic", with ageing. The severity of the disease can be estimated by measuring the bone mineral density (BMD).

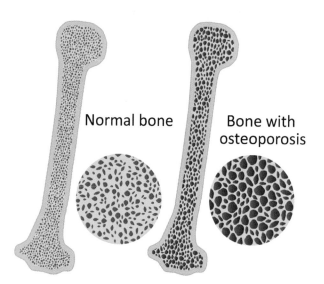
Normal bone   Bone with osteoporosis

Normal bone and osteoporotic bone

Osteopaenia and osteoporosis are more pronounced in women than men, as the decrease of sex hormones in women following menopause increases the chance of developing osteoporosis. Sex hormones are needed to maintain the calcium and protein in the bone. Women who have been through the change and are in menopause have decreased amounts of sex hormones.

Medicines are available to counteract osteoporosis. However, these medicines only decrease the amount of bone removed naturally by the body. The reasoning behind prescribing these medicines is that slowing down the removal of bone would then increase the total amount of bone that is still present.

However, the bad news is that the bone that remains is old. Old bone is not as strong or healthy as fresh new bone. Hence the medicine provided to treat osteoporosis does not produce good new bone. In actual fact, it may even suppress new bone formation.

But the great news is that exercise is different. It creates new bone. The fresh new bone that is formed as a result of exercise is far superior to the retained old bone. Resistance training and weight-bearing activity are effective ways for older adults to maintain and increase the strength of their bones [1]. Hence, exercise acts both as an effective measure to prevent the development of osteoporosis and helps with the treatment for osteoporosis if the condition develops [1].

Hip fractures

Hip fractures are painful and debilitating injuries, especially for older people. Hip fractures are related to osteoporosis. A hip fracture requires a major operation to either fix the broken bone or to replace the

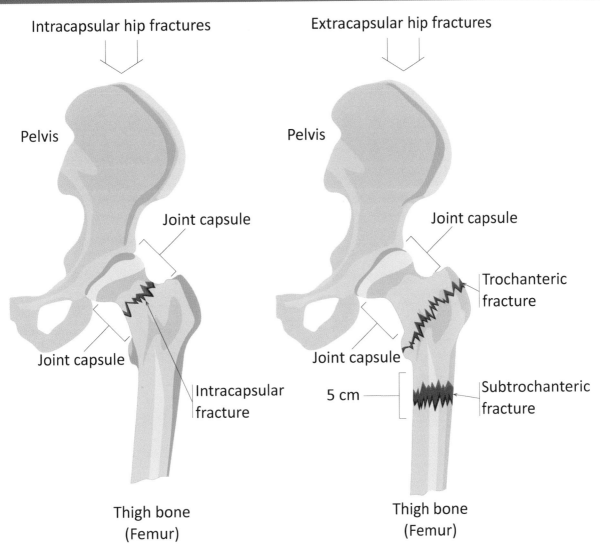

Intracapsular hip fractures

Extracapsular hip fractures

Pelvis

Pelvis

Joint capsule

Joint capsule

Trochanteric fracture

Joint capsule

Joint capsule

Intracapsular fracture

5 cm

Subtrochanteric fracture

Thigh bone (Femur)

Thigh bone (Femur)

The different types of hip fractures

hip. Following such a major operation, it can take many months or up to a year to regain maximum muscle strength and mobility. It is therefore vital to do everything possible to avoid the injury in the first instance.

A paper by researchers Feskanich and team investigated the possible relationship between exercise and hip fracture risk. In this study, the activity levels (including walking, sitting and ten other forms of activity) of 35,996 men aged 50 years and older were observed for a period of 24 years [2]. Feskanich and colleagues used the results of this study to calculate the

relationship between physical activity and the risk of hip fractures. Their most significant finding revealed that simply walking more often lowered the risk of hip fractures by as much as 43% [2].

Walking is a weight-bearing exercise. This means that the bones in the legs carry the weight of the body while walking. The increased weight and stress transmitted to the bones allows the generation of new bone and prevents osteoporosis. The new bone makes the bones strong, and they are less likely to break or fracture even following a fall.

References

1. McMillan LB, Zengin A, Ebeling PR, Scott D. Prescribing Physical Activity for the Prevention and Treatment of Osteoporosis in Older Adults. Healthcare (Basel). 2017;5(4):85. Published 2017 Nov 6.

2. Feskanich D, Flint AJ, Willett WC. Physical activity and inactivity and risk of hip fractures in men. Am J Public Health. 2014;104(4):e75-e81.

Metaphor 3 – Can Weak Muscles Damage My Joints and Discs?

What is the story?
Penelope bought a new car. The manual of the vehicle stated that the tyres required a certain air pressure. Initially, the tyres were well inflated and there were no problems.

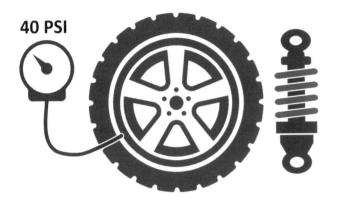

40 PSI

Over time, the tyres began to lose air and became deflated, but Penelope was too busy to go to the garage. She ignored the problem and continued to drive. Driving on the deflated tyres caused the car to become unstable. This instability damaged the shock absorbers in her car.

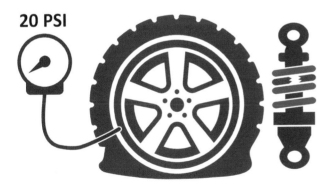

20 PSI

As the shock absorbers were damaged, she had to take her car to the garage to get them replaced and her tyres pumped up.

So, what went wrong?
Penelope did not take good care of her car.

If she had looked after her vehicle and re-inflated the tyres as the manual had instructed, then the car would not have become unstable, and the shock absorbers would not have become damaged.

How can we relate this story to our health?
The muscles in our body are like the car tyres in the story. The discs in the spine and the joints in our limbs are like the shock absorbers. If our muscles are strong, then there is less stress on our discs and joints.

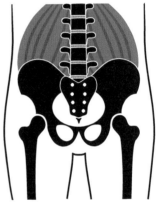

If the muscles are weak, the increased stress will damage and injure our discs and joints. The muscles and the discs/joints are a pair and need to work together.

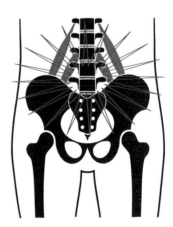

Moral of the story
Muscles and Joints/Discs - United we stand, divided we fall.

Reason 4 – Exercise Improves Muscle Health, Decreases Weight and Combats Obesity

Sarcopenia

Sarcopenia is the loss of muscle mass and strength as we age [1]. This process involves a decline in muscle fibres which begins from the age of 50. It will occur in everyone when they reach a certain age. This will also happen in athletes.

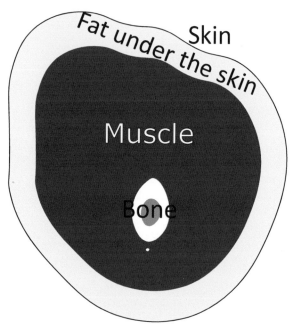

Cross-section of a normal thigh showing an appropriate mix of muscle and fat

However, lack of exercise increases the chances of developing sarcopaenia much more and also decreases the age at which it first presents. Hence, individuals who lead a sedentary lifestyle will lose more strength earlier than those who exercise often [1]. In the UK, sarcopenia affects 4.6% of older men and 7.9% of older women [1].

The resulting loss of muscle mass increases physical disability and causes poor quality of life and early death [1]. In addition, the associated muscle weakness reduces stability and increases the risk of falling and causing injuries. As a result of these negative effects, sarcopenia has become a focal point of research and public debate. Despite this attention, it remains poorly managed in real life [1].

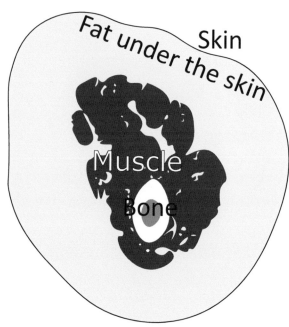

Cross-section of the thigh with sarcopenia showing higher fat to muscle ratio

There are, unfortunately, no medications or injections available to treat the condition. Hence, the management of sarcopenia relies heavily on muscle strengthening exercises [1]. Resistance and strengthening exercises, even performed for short periods of time, can halt the progression of sarcopenia [1].

Obesity

Obesity is a dangerous and prominent problem in today's society. Its prevalence has increased dramatically over the past decades, to the point where it is now considered a global epidemic [2]. Obesity is associated with an increased risk of numerous chronic diseases, including cardiovascular disease, cancer, and osteoarthritis [2]. Consequently, it is also related to an increased risk of disability [2]. Tackling obesity is, therefore, an important task but, unfortunately, is not easily achieved.

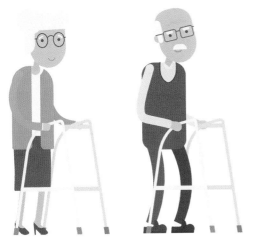

Lack of exercise causes sarcopenia

Exercise alone cannot combat obesity but helps in weight reduction. Exercise needs to be combined with a healthy diet and behavioural changes to reduce weight effectively.

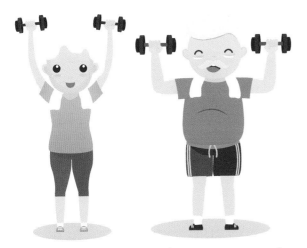

Exercise prevents and cures sarcopenia

A 2019 study by Budui and team assessed the short-term effectiveness of an intensive multi-dimensional rehabilitation program (MRP) on elderly patients with severe obesity [2]. The rehabilitation programme included diet, exercise and behavioural therapy and was conducted for a period of three weeks [2]. The results of the study showed that even after just three weeks of a multi-dimensional rehabilitation programme, the three following changes occurred. On average, body weight reduced by 3.4%, Body Mass Index (BMI) by 3.9% and waist circumference by 3.4% [2]. The study concluded that the three-week multi-dimensional rehabilitation programme provided significant obesity-related improvements. This can, in turn, lead to a reduced risk of obesity-associated conditions, decreased frailty and improved quality of life [2].

The muscle-to-fat ratio
Although obesity is bad for health for numerous reasons, what really matters regarding musculoskeletal pain, is the fat-to-muscle ratio. Consider this metaphor: when constructing a building, a builder needs both cement and sand. It is crucial that the builder has the right mix of cement and sand for the structure to be strong. If there is too much sand and too little cement, the structure will be weak and more likely to fall apart. In the human body, muscle is like the cement and fat is like the sand. It does not matter if a person is large or small; what matters is the right mix of muscle and fat. Too much fat and not enough muscle will weaken the structure of the body, causing pain. Hence, a thin lady with no muscle is more at risk of musculoskeletal pain than a large person with more muscle. Even if a person is overweight, as long as they have a good muscle-to-fat ratio, they could avoid musculoskeletal pain. This highlights the importance of keeping the muscles strong

and avoiding sarcopaenia, whilst managing body fat percentage and evading obesity.

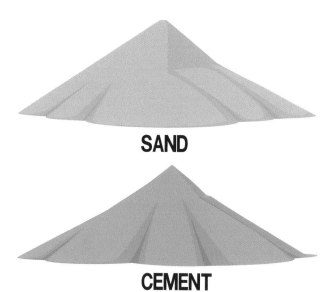

SAND

CEMENT

Every building needs the right mix of sand and cement. Too little cement will make the building weak. Similarly, too little muscle will make the body weak.

Want to test yourself for sarcopaenia?
Complete the SARC-F questionnaire. The SARC-F questionnaire is a brief screening test for sarcopaenia. It is a simple five-item questionnaire that detects if a person is at risk of the condition [3]. The questionnaire has exhibited good reliability and validity [3]. We have included the questionnaire below to enable you to screen yourself for the condition. Answer these five questions and add up your score. A total score of 4 or more indicates sarcopaenia.

1. Strength - How much difficulty do you have in lifting and carrying 10 pounds?
   None = 0
   Some = 1
   A lot or unable = 2

2. Assistance in walking - How much difficulty do you have walking across a room?
   None = 0
   Some = 1
   A lot, use aids, or unable = 2

3. Rise from a chair - How much difficulty do you have transferring from a chair or bed?
   None = 0
   Some = 1
   A lot or unable without help = 2

4. Climb stairs - How much difficulty do you have climbing a flight of ten stairs?
   None = 0
   Some = 1
   A lot or unable = 2

5. Falls - How many times have you fallen in the last year?
   None = 0
   1–3 falls = 1
   4 or more falls = 2

References
1. Dhillon RJ, Hasni S. Pathogenesis and Management of Sarcopenia. Clin Geriatr Med. 2017;33(1):1726.
2. Budui S, Bigolin F, Giordano F, Leoni S, Berteotti M, Sartori E, Franceschini L, Taddei M, Salvetti S, Castiglioni F, Gilli F, Skafidas S, Schena F, Petroni M, L, Busetto L: Effects of an Intensive Inpatient Rehabilitation Program in Elderly Patients with Obesity. Obes Facts 2019;12:199-210.
3. Malmstrom TK, Miller DK, Simonsick EM, Ferrucci L, Morley JE. SARC-F: a symptom score to predict persons with sarcopenia at risk for poor functional outcomes. J Cachexia Sarcopenia Muscle. 2016;7(1):28-36.

Metaphor 4 – Why Does My Back Hurt With Any Movement?

What is the story?
There was a problem with the gearbox in Philip's car. When he started the car, he tried to put it into first gear to move off. Due to the damage in the gearbox, Philip was unable to engage first gear and it automatically slipped into fourth gear. The car then stalled, and Philip was unable to move forward.

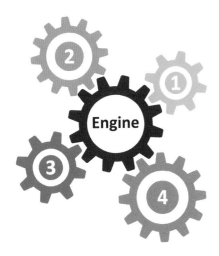

So, what went wrong?
To move off from a stationary position, we initially need to engage the first gear, then the second and so on to the fourth gear. If the gearbox is damaged and the first gear will not engage, we are unlikely to move forward.

How can we relate this story to our health?
Many different layers of muscles surround the spine. Each layer has a specific purpose. The muscle layer closest to the spine "stabilises" the spine and the layers further away "move" the spine. In the ideal situation, the "stabilisers" need to act before the "movers". The "stabiliser" muscles are small and after an injury or a bout of back pain, the "stabiliser" muscles become weak, whilst the "mover" muscles are large and do not. In this situation, the larger "movers" work more to compensate for the weakness in the "stabilisers". When the larger "movers" act without the smaller "stabilisers", it creates abnormal forces across the discs in the spine. This, unfortunately, causes sudden spasms of back pain.

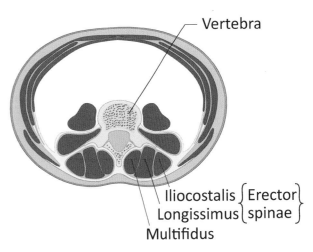

Cross-section of the trunk. The tummy is at the top and the spinal column with the muscles are at the bottom of the figure. The multifidus, the longissimus and the Iliocostalis are the muscles that surround the spinal column.

This is like the gearbox falling into fourth gear when attempting to engage the first gear. In the car, the faulty gearbox can be changed, but the muscles in the back cannot be replaced. The good news, however, is that the "stabilisers" can be retrained to start their action before the "movers". Repeatedly pulling in our belly button towards our spine and pulling up the pelvic sling retrains the smaller "stabilisers".

Moral of the story
Look after the small muscles and the bigger ones will look after themselves.

Reason 5 – Exercise Reduces Risk and Effects of Cancer

The threat of colon, breast, prostate, and lung cancer all increase with age. A lack of adequate activity can further increase this risk and is known to contribute to the development of 2% of all cancers [1]. Conversely, regular exercise has shown to reduce the risk of cancer [1]. This is evident in the review by Brown and colleagues in 2012. In this review, the researchers examined the results of previous studies which had investigated the effects that physical activity and exercise can have on various cancers [1].

Breast cancer

Breast cancer is a major issue and accounts for almost a quarter of all cancers in women [1]. Worldwide, around 1.4 million women are diagnosed with breast cancer each year, and 500,000 die from the disease [1]. Risk factors for the condition include physical inactivity, alcohol consumption and obesity [1]. The review by Brown and team evaluated 73 studies that had examined the association between breast cancer and exercise. They found that regular exercise reduced the overall risk of breast cancer by 20-30% [1]. In addition, they also found that that increasing the duration of physical activity provided greater benefits. Engaging in physical activity for more than six and a half hours a week could reduce the threat of breast cancer by 28%, whilst exercising for only two to three hours only provided a 7% reduction of risk [1].

Even after developing the disease, exercise seems to help. Patients undergoing treatment for breast cancer may have trouble sleeping. Exercise has been found to improve the sleep quality in these patients. Exercise also seems to increase the patients' chances of completing chemotherapy [2].

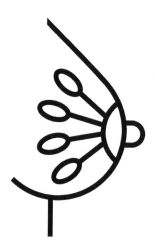

Colon cancer

Colon cancer is cancer of the large bowel. Annually, it is diagnosed in around 1.2 million people around the world, and 600,000 die as a result of the disease each year [1]. Surgical treatment for the condition may involve removing the bowel and having an external colostomy bag fitted. Diet and lifestyle, including physical inactivity, are identified as risk factors for developing colon cancer [1].

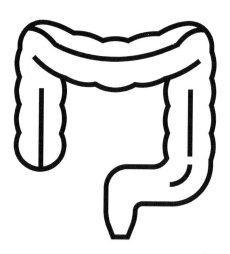

Brown's review showed that regular exercise and leisure time activity could reduce the risk of colon cancer by almost 25% [1]. Just like in breast cancer, more exercise equalled greater risk reductions [1]. Even after developing the disease, exercise seems to decrease recurrence or the chance of the disease coming back [2].

Prostate cancer

Worldwide, over 900,000 men are diagnosed with prostate cancer each year and the risk factors include a sedentary lifestyle and obesity [1]. The review by Brown showed that physical activity decreased the risk of developing prostate cancer by 10% [1].

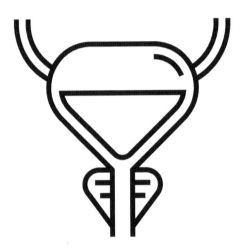

In addition, after developing the disease, men find that the treatment increases fatigue and decreases their sex drive. Fortunately, exercise can combat these side effects, allowing patients to remain physically and sexually active as they undergo prostate cancer treatment [2].

Pancreatic cancer

The pancreas is an organ within the abdomen that regulates blood sugar and aids in digestion. Pancreatic cancer is difficult to beat. Only 4% of people diagnosed with the disease survive for five years after receiving their diagnosis [1]. Brown and colleagues found that the

individuals with high levels of physical activity reduced their risk of pancreatic cancer by 28% as compared to others who were not physically active [1].

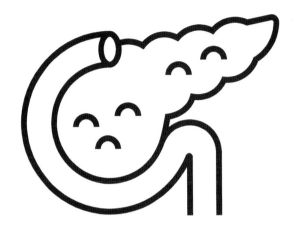

Lung cancer

Worldwide, 1.2 million people are diagnosed with lung cancer each year and almost 1 million lung cancer patients die annually [1]. The review of Brown and colleagues showed that physical activity reduced the risk of lung cancer by 23-38% and the reductions were dependent on the intensity of the exercise [1]. Physical activity also improves the psychological and physical well-being of individuals who were undergoing treatment [2].

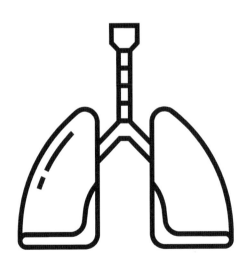

References

1. Brown JC, Winters-Stone K, Lee A, Schmitz KH. Cancer, physical activity, and exercise. Compr Physiol. 2012;2(4):2775-2809.

2. Luan X, Tian X, Zhang H, Huang R, Li N, Chen P, Wang R. Exercise as a prescription for patients with various diseases. J Sport Health Sci. 2019 Sep;8(5):422-44.

Metaphor 5 – Who Has a Greater Role to Play?

What is the story?

Pablo and Parker were seven-year-old twin boys. Peter, their father, was very keen for the boys to try for the school football team, so he signed them for football training.

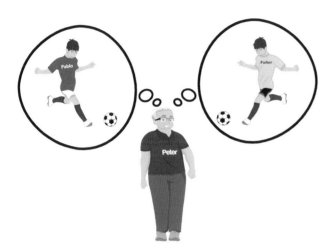

Parker was eager to train and regularly attended practice. He played football whenever he could find some spare time.

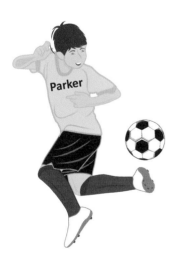

Pablo did not want to put any extra time into football and much preferred to watch T.V. instead.

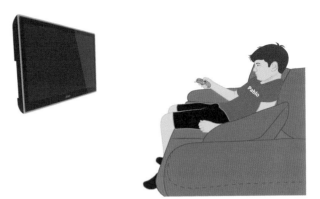

Parker made it onto the team at the football trials thanks to all his hard work, but Pablo did not, leaving him disappointed.

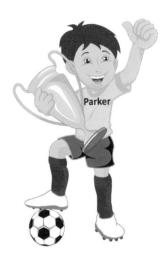

So, what went wrong?

Pablo and Parker both had access to the same resources to help to improve their football abilities, but only Parker chose to take advantage of this. Parker took ownership and devoted his own time to training. Pablo decided not to spend any extra time practising and as a result, was unable to make it onto the team.

How can we relate this story to our health?
To improve our health, we must take ownership of the issue. Just as the boys had access to classes, we have access to exercises to improve our health. The point is that we must actively choose to participate and spend time on these things. We cannot rely solely on health care professionals. Only we can strengthen our muscles by taking ownership of wanting to improve our health. Healthcare professionals are only there to guide us on how to achieve our goals.

Moral of the story
Hard work pays off when improving our health.

Reason 6 – Exercise Reduces the Effects of Alzheimer's Disease (AD) and Combats Depression

Alzheimer's

Alzheimer's is the most common type of memory loss, accounting for 60-80% of cases [1]. It starts as a mild cognitive impairment. However, in more than half of the cases, it develops into Alzheimer's disease (AD) within five years [1]. Alzheimer's progressively destroys memory and thinking skills, including executive function. Executive function refers to a set of mental skills that consist of working memory, self-control, and mental flexibility. These skills are essential in life and are used in many daily tasks. Hence, their destruction as a result of Alzheimer's disease can significantly reduce a person's quality of life. Furthermore, patients with Alzheimer's often experience agitation, anxiety, depression and injury. Drug treatment can help, but the benefits can be limited [1].

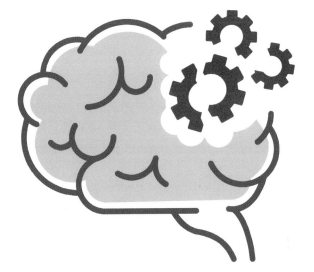

Aerobic exercises seem to decrease the onset of mild cognitive impairment and Alzheimer's disease. It also reduces the rate of deterioration once the disease process has commenced. Exercise has shown to improve attention, executive function, memory, processing speed and blood flow.

A small part of the brain called the hippocampus is involved in memory. There is a decay of the hippocampus in patients with Alzheimer's disease. Exercise seems to increase the blood supply and decrease the decay in the hippocampus. MRI scans have verified this.

Another effect of exercise on Alzheimer's disease is through nerve factors. Brain-derived neurotrophic factor is one of the proteins that maintain brain function. This is decreased in Alzheimer's disease. Exercise seems to maintain levels of this nerve factor which then prevents reduction in the volume of the brain.

Want to test yourself / someone for signs of dementia?

The following test [2] is used across the UK to help investigate cognitive decline in a primary care setting (for example at the GP). It would be best to do this test with someone else guiding you through, so that they can check the accuracy of your answers. If you do complete this test with any mistakes, do not worry – you can go and talk to your GP if you have any further questions about this.

There are 6 questions as part of this assessment – with each question weighted differently. The scoring is detailed below.

To complete this assessment, ask the individual the following questions:

1. What year is it? (Correct = 0 points. Incorrect = 4 points)

2. What month is it? (Correct = 0 points. Incorrect = 3 points)

3. Give the person an address phrase to remember with 5 components – e.g. John, Smith, 42, High St, Bedford

4. About what time is it (within one hour)? (Correct = 0 points. Incorrect = 3 points)

5. Count backwards from 20 to 1. (Correct = 0 points. 1 error = 2 points. More than one error = 4 points)

6. Say the months of the year in reverse. (Correct = 0 points. 1 error = 2 points. More than one error = 4 points)

7. Repeat address phrase. (Correct = 0 points. 1 error = 2 points. 2 errors = 4 points. 3 errors – 6 points. 4 errors = 8 points. All wrong = 10 points)

To score the individual, add all the scores together to cumulate a total 6CIT score out of 28. Scores of 0-7 are considered normal, with a score of 8 or more being significant.

Depression
Depression is a growing health concern, affecting 264 million people globally [3]. It can be common in older adults and may increase their risk of death from other illnesses, including diabetes and cardiovascular disease. Additionally, depression can sadly result in suicide, causing the loss of valuable lives [3]. Currently, traditional treatments for depression do not yield satisfactory outcomes [3]. Fortunately, there is an abundance of evidence supporting exercise as an effective intervention [3]. For example, a review by researchers Zemberi

and colleagues analysed the results of 13 previous studies. Each of these studies had investigated the efficacy of exercise as the primary intervention for depression [3]. The results of these studies indicated that aerobic exercise (brisk walking, running etc.) and high-intensity progressive resistance training (PRT) were effective in reducing depressive symptoms and their severity [3].

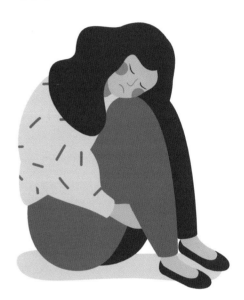

Exercise also seems to enhance the effect of anti-depressants. The combined effect of exercise with anti-depressants is greater than the sum total of the individual effects [3].

References
1. Meng Q, Lin MS, Tzeng IS. Relationship Between Exercise and Alzheimer's Disease: A Narrative Literature Review. Front Neurosci. 2020;14:131. Published 2020 Mar 26.
2. Velayudhan L, Ryu SH, Raczek M, Philpot M, Lindesay J, Critchfield M, Livingston G. Review of brief cognitive tests for patients with suspected dementia. Int Psychogeriatr. 2014 Aug;26(8):1247-62. .

3. Md Zemberi NFN, Ismail MM, Abdullah
    MFIL. Exercise Interventions as the
    Primary Treatment for Depression:
    Evidence from a Narrative
    Review. Malays J Med Sci. 2020;27(5):5

Metaphor 6 – "Credit Limit" is Like "Activity Limit"

What is the story?
Patrick's business had a downturn, and he became bankrupt. He needed a credit card but found it challenging to find one due to his poor financial status. In the end, one bank manager gave him a credit card with only a £200 credit limit.

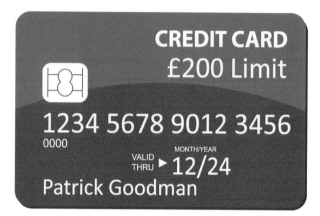

Patrick knew that he would be fined if he went over this limit. Patrick was careful to spend only £190 of the available £200 to be well under the limit.

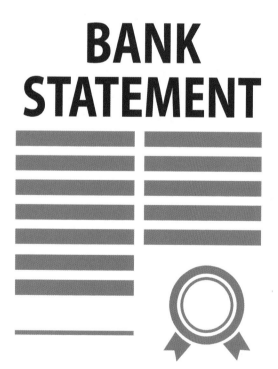

After remaining well under his limit for a few months, the bank manager increased the credit limit to £250. For the next few months, Patrick spent up to £240 to make sure he was well under the new limit. Over time, Patrick slowly but surely built up his business and increased his credit limit, becoming very successful. If he had gone over the limit, then he would have been fined and the credit facility would have been removed.

So, what went wrong?
Well, nothing went wrong in this story. Patrick respected the limits put on him by his bank manager. He remained well under these limits and as a result, over time, his limits were increased, and he was able to build up his credit and business.

How can we relate this story to our health?
When we have chronic pain, our brain gives us an "activity limit". The "activity limit" is the "pain barrier". This "activity limit" is similar to the "credit limit" given to Patrick. If we go beyond the "activity limit", the inner brain will cause pain, just as the bank manager would have fined Patrick if he had gone over the "credit limit".

Patrick stayed well within the "credit limit" and found that the "credit limit" was increased automatically with time. Similarly, when we exercise following injury, we need to stay within the "activity limit" determined by our inner brain. Note that Patrick never spent beyond £190 of the £200 limit or £240 of his £250 limit. Similarly, it is best to keep well within the "activity limit". If we respect the limits given to us by our brain and stick to the traffic light system described in the introduction of this book, then, over time, we can do more and more.

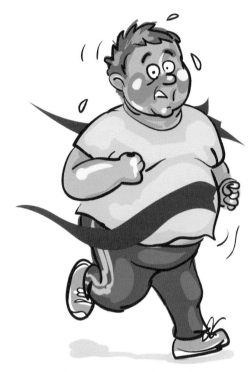

Do not break/fight the pain barrier

Moral of the story
In chronic pain (or following injury) - don't fight the pain barrier.

Reason 7 – Exercise Reduces Inflammation, Heart Attacks, Strokes and Chronic Obstructive Pulmonary Disease (COPD)

Inflammation

During physical activity, the muscles release proteins called myokines. Myokines were only identified in 2003. These proteins are only released when the muscles contract or become active. It does not get secreted when the muscles are resting. Myokines can be thought of as a magical substance that gets secreted when the body exercises. All the beneficial effects of the myokines are still not known. More and more are being identified by ongoing research. However, they play a major role in decreasing inflammation, improving metabolism, and regulating the immune system. Decreasing inflammation helps with heart disease and diabetes. Myokines are also known to inhibit tumour formation and improve brain function. Myokines are released even with a single bout of exercise [1].

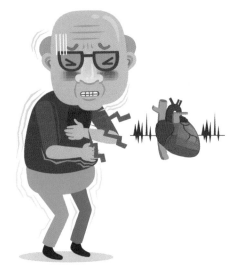

Narrowing and partial blockage of the blood vessel to the heart causes angina. Complete blockage of the blood vessel causes a myocardial infarction (heart attack).

Cardiovascular Disease (CVD) and Strokes

Cardiovascular disease (CVD) refers to conditions affecting the heart and blood vessels. Genetics, diet and a lack of exercise promote the development of plaques within the arteries. Blood clots may form around the plaque and decrease or stop the blood supply to the heart. When the blood supply to the heart is reduced, the condition is called angina. When the blood supply to part of the heart is completely cut off or blocked, it is called a myocardial infarction or a heart attack.

When the blood supply to part of the brain is completely cut off or blocked, then the condition is called a cerebrovascular accident or stroke.

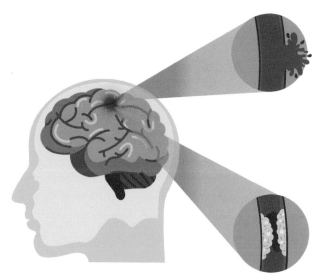

A cerebrovascular accident, or a stroke, occurs when the blood vessel to the brain becomes completely blocked or bursts, causing bleeding.

Cardiovascular disease is seen in more than one in three adults [2]. Over half of these cases are in people over the age of 60 [2]. Fortunately, exercise can be beneficial. Soares-Miranda and team investigated this in their 2016 study. They observed 4,207 men and women, with an average age of

73, for a period of ten years [2]. At the start of the study, all participants were free of cardiovascular disease. The researchers assessed each of the participant's activity levels (including walking, leisure time activity and exercise intensity) throughout the duration of the study and observed any cardiovascular disease events. They found that greater physical activity was associated with a lower risk of coronary heart disease (the leading cause of heart attacks) and stroke, even in participants aged 75 years and older [2]. The study concluded that physical activity, in particular walking, should be recommended to reduce the incidence of cardiovascular disease among older adults [2].

COPD

Chronic obstructive pulmonary disease (COPD) is a term used to describe a class of inflammatory lung conditions that cause obstruction of airflow into and out of the lungs.

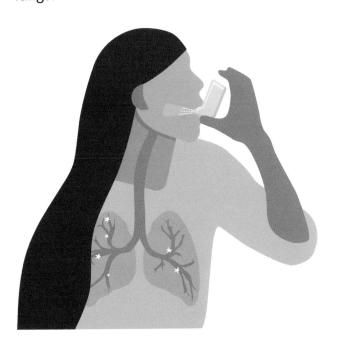

COPD causes difficulty breathing and patients may need inhalers

To treat individuals with COPD, a supervised program called pulmonary rehabilitation is often prescribed. This programme includes exercise training and health education and has been shown to provide benefits [3]. A review by Jenkins and team analysed six trials, which included a total of 790 patients with chronic obstructive pulmonary disease. These trials compared supervised maintenance exercise programmes with usual care (no extra treatment) following pulmonary rehabilitation [3]. These trials showed that continued supervised exercise significantly reduced the risk of hospital admissions caused by respiratory problems. They also found that this additional care reduced the risk of death by almost 50% [3].

References

1. Bay ML, Pedersen BK. Muscle-Organ Crosstalk: Focus on Immunometabolism. Front Physiol. 2020;11:567881. Published 2020 Sep 9.
2. Soares-Miranda L, Siscovick DS, Psaty BM, Longstreth WT Jr, Mozaffarian D. Physical Activity and Risk of Coronary Heart Disease and Stroke in Older Adults: The Cardiovascular Health Study. Circulation. 2016;133(2):147-155.
3. Jenkins AR, Gowler H, Curtis F, Holden NS, Bridle C, Jones AW. Efficacy of supervised maintenance exercise following pulmonary rehabilitation on health care use: a systematic review and meta-analysis. Int J Chron Obstruct Pulmon Dis. 2018;13:257-273.

Metaphor 7 – Can Steroid Injections Cure Me?

What is the story?
Patterson was very hungry and had two options. He could go down to the vending machine and buy a fizzy drink and a chocolate bar, or he could go to the canteen and buy a salad and a bottle of water.

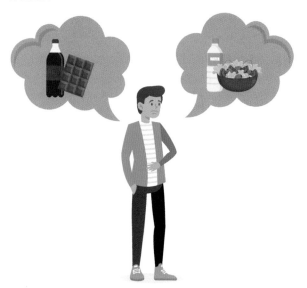

Patterson decided to opt for the chocolate bar and drink. An hour later, he felt hungry again.

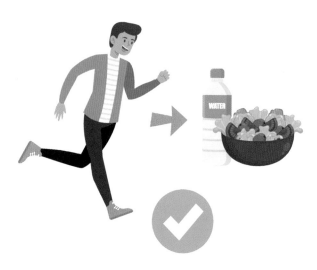

So, what went wrong?
When we are hungry, it can be easy to

think that the sugary treat will help. Unfortunately, this will only give us a "sugar rush". Foods such as these will keep us full for only 30 minutes and we are unlikely to get the energy over a long period. On the other hand, a full meal, whilst seeming more time-consuming, will keep us fuelled and energetic for longer.

How can we relate this story to our health?
When we experience pain, we have a choice about which treatment option to choose. For instance, we can go for the more long-term option, such as muscle-strengthening exercises. Alternatively, we can choose to go for the quick option, such as steroid injections as a form of short-term pain relief. There is a time and place for quick options such as steroid injections. However, there is only so much good that injections can do. Studies have shown that steroid injections may have adverse effects on the strength and stability of the muscles. Exercises and constant work may seem like a harder option, but often, it is more effective in the long term.

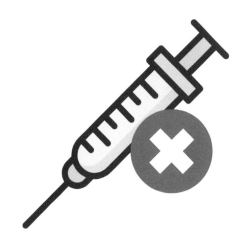

Moral of the story
In pain – a quick fix is only a short fix.

Reason 8 – Exercise Makes You Live Longer and Does Not Cause Harm

Exercise and increased longevity

With all the health benefits that come with physical activity, the most sought after is increased longevity. It is the goal of most people to live a long and happy life, and exercise can play a vital role in achieving this. However, as people age, they may be less inclined to partake in physical activity. This is detrimental to health and the pursuit of longevity. A study in 2011 by Xue and team examined 433 initially high-functioning older women aged 70-79 years old over 12 years [1]. All the participants were categorised into four different groups according to the level of their regular physical activity [1].

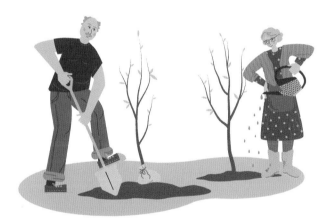

Routine household tasks like gardening were helpful

The four groups were as follows: always active, fast-declining (meaning their physical activity is on a steep decline) stable-moderate (meaning their activity levels are moderate but stable), and always-sedentary [1]. The research looked at four exercise activities and two lifestyle activities. The exercise activities were walking, dancing, bowling, and strengthening exercises. The two lifestyle

activities were strenuous household activity, like scrubbing and outdoor activity, like gardening. Increased risk of various conditions, including coronary artery disease, obesity, depression and chronic obstructive pulmonary disease, was associated with sedentary behaviour and/or a fast decline in activity [1]. This shows that a sudden decrease in the level of the activity needs to be monitored. Other factors including low self-belief, disability, and low energy were also associated with an increased risk of developing various health disorders [1].

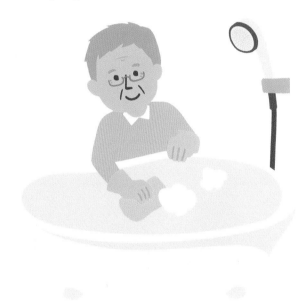

Routine household tasks like scrubbing and cleaning were also helpful

Additionally, women in the always-sedentary classification were over three times more likely to die than women from the always-active group [1]. Surprisingly, both the groups in the moderately-active and always-active did well. This showed that exercise does not have to be intense to be beneficial [1]. These results indicate that people who remain active in their later years increase their chances of survival significantly whilst reducing the threat of numerous health conditions. The most important finding is that routine and simple activities like walking, scrubbing and gardening helped to achieve this superior health status.

Exercise does not cause harm

Whilst running is known to have many health benefits, including improvements in cardiovascular fitness and longevity, controversy exists regarding the harm running can cause to the knees. It has been previously theorised that running may cause damage to the knee joints, promoting the development of conditions such as osteoarthritis (OA). However, this is now generally viewed as a misconception.

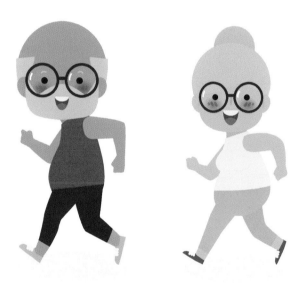

Running does not cause arthritis in the joints

A study in 2017 by Lo and colleagues attempted to find evidence regarding this. The study consisted of 2,637 female participants aged 45 to 79 years [2]. The researchers observed the symptoms, investigation findings and lifetime physical activity surveys in order to examine the relationship between running history and incidence of knee osteoarthritis. The study

concluded that there was no increased risk of symptomatic knee osteoarthritis among runners as compared with non-runners [2]. The findings of this study indicate that running has little to no effect on the condition of the knees, or the occurrence of knee osteoarthritis, over the course of a lifetime.

References

1. Xue QL, Bandeen-Roche K, Mielenz TJ, et al. Patterns of 12-year change in physical activity levels in community-dwelling older women: can modest levels of physical activity help older women live longer?. Am J Epidemiol. 2012;176(6):534-543.
2. Lo GH, Driban JB, Kriska AM, et al. Is There an Association Between a History of Running and Symptomatic Knee Osteoarthritis? A Cross-Sectional Study From the Osteoarthritis Initiative. Arthritis Care Res (Hoboken). 2017;69(2):183-191.

Metaphor 8 – A Stitch in Time Saves Nine

What is the story?
Prem is a junior executive. He has to make an important presentation to the board in the afternoon. He noticed a small hole in his trousers in the morning, but it wasn't visible, so he chose to ignore it and went to work.

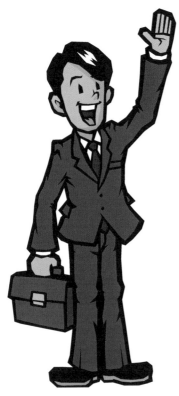

He was in for a promotion and would get to lead the project if he did well. Unfortunately, just before the meeting, as he bent down to pick some files from off the floor, his trousers ripped badly. He had no spare trousers and could not go in front of the board with the damaged ones. Another colleague substituted for him and presented the project. This colleague was promoted and was made the project leader. Prem, despite his hard work, was not rewarded.

So, what went wrong?
Prem chose to ignore the initial damage to his trousers. Unfortunately, a small bit of damage, when not fixed initially, can become a big problem. If he had fixed the trousers initially, they might not have ripped so badly that they became unwearable.

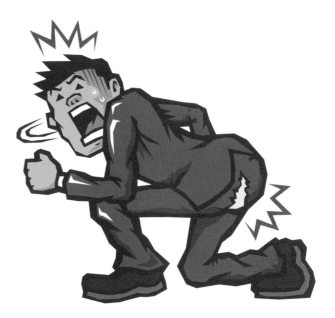

How can we relate this story to our health?
When we first notice a back injury, we may be tempted to ignore it and not move that body part, believing it will sort itself out. However, not moving the body part makes the muscles weaker. Weaker muscles can transfer greater stress onto the disc and joints. Increased stress to the disc can cause a disc to prolapse. Increased stress to the joint can cause wear and tear. It is important to slowly but surely keep active, and exercise even when the problem is only minor.

Moral of the story
With a small initial injury - a stitch in time saves nine.

Reason 9 – Exercise Aids Compression of Morbidity and Decreases Frailty

In the last century, developed countries have seen life expectancy increase by over 30 years [1]. This increase in life expectancy is also seen in developing countries but at a slower pace. The challenge now is to ensure that this essentially new lease of life is not plagued by disability or illness. Unfortunately, the last part of life before death is often spent in frailty and disability. The goal is to shorten this period of frailty and disability. This is called "compression of morbidity". Components of this frailty and disability include muscle weakness, slowed walking (gait), low physical activity, fatigue and exhaustion and unintentional weight loss.

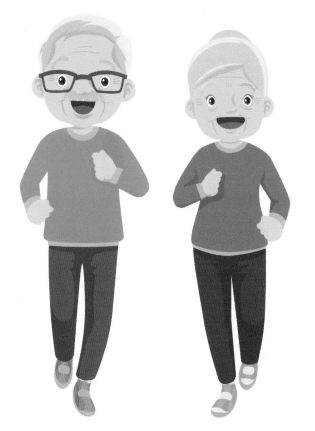

Exercise makes the muscles more youth-like

Studies have shown that exercise and activity delay the onset of frailty [1]. On the contrary, seniors who are sedentary have longer periods of frailty or morbidity. They have illnesses and need care for longer periods.

Research has shown that the muscle tissue of seniors who are involved in regular exercise is similar to that of young adults. It seems muscle is the key organ that shortens or lengthens frailty in later life. If the muscles are strong and keep on working, then the period of disability and frailty prior to passing away is short. But if the muscles are weak and are not involved in regular exercise, then the period of disability and frailty prior to passing away is lengthened.

As exercise can maintain muscle tissue, it can therefore prevent seniors from becoming frail.

Another indicator associated with contributing to frailty is elevated glucose levels in the blood [1]. Generally, frail seniors have high glucose levels and non-frail seniors have lower glucose levels. This may be just because of exercise. Research shows that 150 minutes of physical activity per week works better than medications in reducing blood glucose [1]. In summary, exercise seems like the key component for decreasing frailty in seniors, and therefore aiding in the compression of morbidity.

Running and compression of morbidity.
A study published in 2011 investigated the effects running can have on the compression of morbidity. The study was conducted over a 21-year period. Participants over the age of 50, including

both runners and non-runners, were recruited in 1984. There were 538 runners with 423 healthy control subjects who did not run. At entry and every year thereafter, participants were asked to complete the Health Assessment Questionnaire Disability Index (HAQ-DI) to determine their physical ability. This questionnaire asked participants to report how difficult they found everyday tasks including dressing, walking, and eating. They were required to score each activity out of 3 (0 = no difficulty, 3 = unable to perform). Participants also reported their exercise habits once a year throughout the 21-year study period [2]. Every time data was collected, scores on the HAQ-ID were higher for non-runners than runners (i.e., disability was greater in non-runners than runners) [2]. This suggests that running helped maintain the physical ability of runners throughout the study.

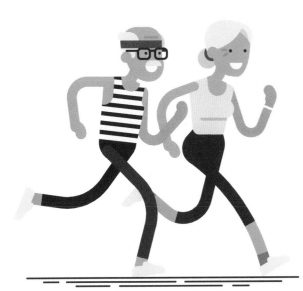

If you are over 50 and run regularly, the chance of you needing a hip or knee replacement is decreased.

Furthermore, during the study the disability scores for both groups increased with age. However, this increase was slower in runners, who took longer to reach the same levels of disability than non-runners [2]. This indicates that running reduces the progression of disability, thereby aiding in the compression of morbidity. It is also worth noting that, at the 19-year point of the study, only 15% or runners had died, compared to a significant 34% of non-runners [2]. In addition, runners had a decreased need to have a knee or hip replacement. The worry and anxiety of every exercise enthusiast is that the increased exercise will cause the joints to wear out. This study, however, proved otherwise as runners had fewer knee and hip replacements.

References
1. Fried LP. Interventions for Human Frailty: Physical Activity as a Model. Cold Spring Harb Perspect Med. 2016;6(6).
2. Chakravarty EF, Hubert HB, Lingala VB, Fries JF. Reduced disability and mortality among aging runners: a 21-year longitudinal study [published correction appears in Arch Intern Med. 2008 Dec 8;168(22):2496]. Arch Intern Med. 2008;168(15):1638-1646.

Metaphor 9 – Surgery - Is It Worth the Risk?

What is the story?
Percy wants to move from the roof of one tall building to the roof of another tall building. The buildings are about five feet apart. Percy has two options. The first option would be to jump from the roof of one building to the other. The second option would be to climb down one building, cross over on ground level and climb up the other building. The first option seems very easy and quick, but if he misses, there are significant consequences. The second option is slow and protracted, but the risks are minimal. In this situation, Percy would have to weigh up the benefits and risks and decide to either take the short route with higher risks or the long route with fewer risks.

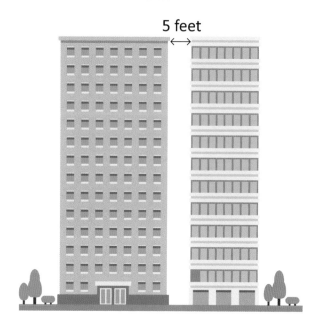

5 feet

So, what went wrong?
Nothing went wrong. Surgery may seem a quick and easy option, but the consequences could be disastrous if things go wrong.

How can we relate this story to our health?
Many of the surgeries performed in Orthopaedics are for wear and tear, which is a natural ageing process. The body part is not broken; it has only suffered some wear and tear. There are specific situations where surgical intervention for wear and tear will help, but surgery is not always effective. Some surgical interventions, like spinal surgery, have a high failure rate. Following spinal surgery, one in five patients go on to develop a condition called "Failed Back Surgery Syndrome". This results in pain that is even more severe than what was experienced before, with no easy means of a cure. Patients who develop this condition sometimes state that they would not have had the surgery in the first place had they had known the potential consequences. Like Percy should have done, patients who consent to undergo surgery should understand the risks and that the surgical procedure itself is irreversible. Although the reward might seem to be a quick and easy outcome, the risks sometimes far outweigh the potential benefits.

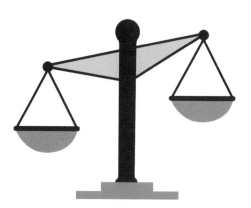

Moral of the story
Be cautious if the risks are high.

Reason 10 – Exercise Decreases Effects of Arthritis and Reduces the Need for Surgery

The most common type of arthritis is called osteoarthritis. In severe cases, it can cause chronic pain, physical disability, and reduced quality of life [1, 2]. Unfortunately, there is no cure for the condition; hence medical treatment is based on symptom reduction. The good news is that exercise can both protect the joint and prevent deterioration once arthritis sets in. It can also decrease the pain and effects of arthritis.

A review by Fransen and team investigated the effects of exercise regarding hip osteoarthritis [1]. They identified nine different research studies which showed that exercise reduced pain and improved physical function in patients with hip osteoarthritis [1]. Their research showed that exercise reduced pain by 8 points on a 0 to 100 scale. On a second 0-100 scale, exercise improved physical function by 7 points [1].

Total Hip Replacement

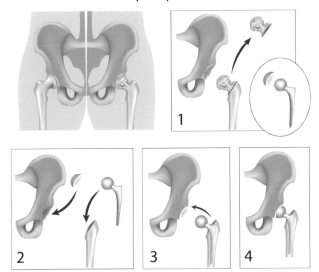

Exercise helps with osteoarthritis of the hip and decreases the need for a total hip replacement

A second review by Fransen and a different team investigated the effects of exercise on knee osteoarthritis [2]. In this review, the researchers identified 44 trials that had obtained evidence suggesting that exercise reduced pain and improved physical function in patients with knee osteoarthritis [2]. On a scale of 0-100, exercise reduced pain by an average of 12 points. On a second 0-100 scale, exercise improved physical function by 10 points [2]. The researchers also identified 13 trials that showed exercise improved overall quality of life for people with knee osteoarthritis [2].

Exercise decreases the onset of the severe symptoms of arthritis

Unfortunately, osteoarthritis is also called "wear and tear" arthritis. This implies that using the joint will increase the "wear and tear" and worsen the symptoms of osteoarthritis. This causes patients with osteoarthritis not to use the joint because of the concern that it could make it worse. This is, however, not the case. Earlier in Reason 8, we showed evidence on how running would reduce the incidence of osteoarthritis. Here, we will show you evidence of how even after a person develops osteoarthritis, running can decrease the symptoms of osteoarthritis. A 2018 study by Lo and team evaluated the association between running and the symptoms of osteoarthritis in the knee [3]. This was similar to the 2017 study by the same research team described in Reason 8. However, rather than investigating the effects of running on the occurrence of osteoarthritis symptoms, they focused on the effects running may have on knees already affected by osteoarthritis. The study included 1203 participants over the age of 50 who had osteoarthritis in at least one knee [3]. Participants who were runners were identified [3] and grouped together. The participants were followed for a period of four years. Outcomes including "worsening knee pain", "new knee pain", and "improved knee pain" were measured [3]. Interestingly, runners made fewer reports of worsening knee pain than non-runners. They were also found to have developed fewer new cases of knee pain throughout the duration of the study [3]. Additionally, runners also experienced higher rates of resolved knee pain than non-runners [3]. This study has clearly shown that running improves pain and symptoms in patients with already-established osteoarthritis of the knee. Hence running should not be discouraged in people with osteoarthritis of the knee [3].

Total Knee Replacement

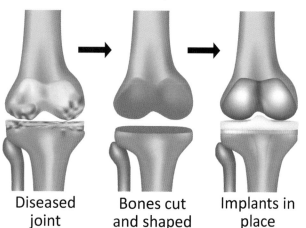

Diseased joint   Bones cut and shaped   Implants in place

Exercise helps with osteoarthritis of the knee and decreases the need for a total knee replacement

Exercise reduces the need for surgical treatment and helps patients who are unable to undergo surgery due to other reasons

It is generally accepted that osteoarthritis is a debilitating condition, which can only get progressively worse over time. In patients with end-stage osteoarthritis of the knee, a total knee replacement (TKR) is often performed to reduce symptoms and improve the quality of life. In recent years there has been a rapid increase in the number of total knee replacements year by year [4].

However, approximately 20% of patients who undergo a total knee replacement still experience long-term pain after surgery [4]. Additionally, as is the case with any surgical procedure, a total knee replacement comes with risks of infection and nerve damage.

Furthermore, some people may not be able to undergo surgery, as they may have other health problems like heart failure, diabetes, or some other condition that prevents them from undergoing surgery. Exercise is a suitable and relatively risk-free option for them.

A study by Skou and team investigated and compared the two-year outcomes of Total Knee Replacements versus non-surgical treatment [4]. All the patients included in the trial were patients who had osteoarthritis and were waiting for knee replacement surgery. The non-surgical treatment included the use of exercise, patient education and insoles. After two years of intervention, the researchers found that the non-surgical treatment improved pain and function in patients with osteoarthritis of the knee [4]. In their study, two-thirds of the patients who were eligible and were informed that they needed a total knee replacement delayed their need for surgery by at least two years [4]. This suggests that patients considering a total knee replacement could first attempt non-surgical interventions, as this may delay their need for the procedure. It is important to talk to your doctor or surgeon and seek their advice. The results of the same research study show that patients who are not suitable for surgery due to other health reasons improved with exercise and found relief from the symptoms of knee osteoarthritis even though they have not been able to undergo surgery [4].

References

1. Fransen M, McConnell S, Hernandez-Molina G, Reichenbach S. Exercise for osteoarthritis of the hip. Cochrane Database Syst Rev. 2009;(3). :CD007912. Published 2009 Jul 8.

2. Fransen M, McConnell S, Harmer AR, Van der Esch M, Simic M, Bennell KL. Exercise for osteoarthritis of the knee: a Cochrane systematic review. Br J Sports Med. 2015;49(24):1554-1557.

3. Lo GH, Musa SM, Driban JB, et al. Running does not increase symptoms or structural progression in people with knee osteoarthritis: data from the osteoarthritis initiative. Clin Rheumatol. 2018;37(9):2497-2504.

4. Skou ST, Roos EM, Laursen MB, Rathleff MS, Arendt-Nielsen L, Rasmussen S, Simonsen O. Total knee replacement and non-surgical treatment of knee osteoarthritis: 2-year outcome from two parallel randomized controlled trials. Osteoarthritis Cartilage. 2018 Sep;26(9):1170-1180.

Metaphor 10 – Showers Don't Clean Your Teeth

What is the story?
Parry was a bus driver and worked long hours. The job was tiring, and he was usually exhausted at the end of a shift. The work was manual and involved turning a heavy steering wheel. He assumed that the heavy work that he was involved in was giving him enough exercise for his entire body.

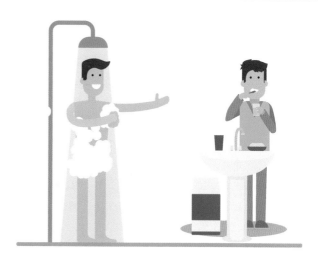

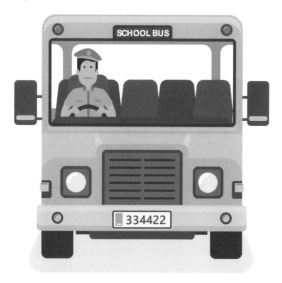

One day, he developed severe back and leg pain. He was diagnosed with sciatica.

So, what went wrong?
Parry wrongly assumed that regular work provided adequate exercise for his whole body. This, unfortunately, is not true. Parry exerted his arms when turning the steering wheel and exerted his legs when operating the foot pedals. There was, however, no exercise for his lower back. Parry's back was weak, and that caused the back pain and sciatica.

How can we relate this story to our health?
Assuming that driving a bus for extended periods will exercise every part of the body is like thinking that a shower will also clean the teeth. Showers do not make our teeth clean, and a separate action of brushing the teeth is required. In the same way, it is crucial that even if we are regularly working, we need to specifically focus on the core muscles in the back to keep it strong and healthy. We tend to exercise our arms and legs more than our core. Not exercising our core, like in Parry's case, can lead to back and spinal problems.

Moral of the story
Don't neglect your core – wrong assumptions can cause harm.

Reason 11 – Exercise Prevents Falls

Falls and fall-related injuries in older people

Falls and fall-related injuries are significant issues in the older population. At least one-third of community-dwelling people over the age of 65 fall each year and the rate of fall-related injuries increases with age [1]. These injuries can be serious, with around 10% of falls resulting in a fracture. Fall-related fractures can cause serious suffering and may even contribute to early death in older adults [1]. Falls can also have various psychological effects on older people, increasing their fear of falling and damaging their confidence. As a result, individuals who have experienced a fall may limit their physical activity, affecting their social life and physical ability [1].

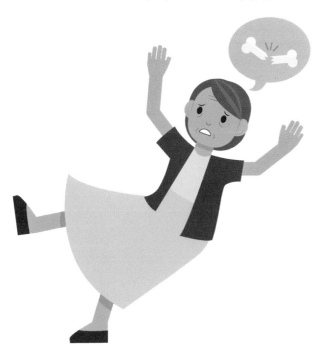

Exercise decreases the risk of falls by 23%

Exercise helps in reducing falls

A review by Sherrington and team investigated the beneficial effect of exercise in reducing falls. They analysed the results of 81 trials which included 19,684 participants and found that exercise reduced the risk of falls by about 23 % [1].

Types of exercise programmes that help reduce falls

The Otago Exercise Programme (OEP) is a home-based exercise programme that was developed in Otago, New Zealand, by Robertson and Campbell. The programme contains strength and balance exercises, which was initially designed to improve stability and coordination in the elderly to reduce falls [2]. The original study recruited 233 participants. The Otago Programme was prescribed to 116 community-dwelling women aged 80 and over [2]. The control group consisted of 117 women of the same age group who were prescribed standard care. After one year of intervention, there were 88 falls in the group of women who exercised compared to 152 falls in the group of women who only received standard care [2]. On average, women who were in the Otago Exercise Programme group only fell 0.8 times during the one-year period, whereas those who only received standard care fell an average of 1.3 times [2]. In addition, the Otago group reduced their risk of fall-related injury by almost 40% and improved their balance scores significantly as compared to those in the group who received standard care [2]. The study concluded that the Otago Exercise Programme improved physical function (balance), reduced the risk of falls and decreased fall-related injuries in women over 80 [2].

Tai chi is a popular form of Chinese martial arts practised for meditation, defence, and health purposes. It involves slow dance-like movements and deep breathing. As Tai chi is a form of low-intensity exercise, it is suitable for older adults. Tai chi has been shown to be effective in improving dynamic and one-legged balance, as well as aiding in fall prevention [3].

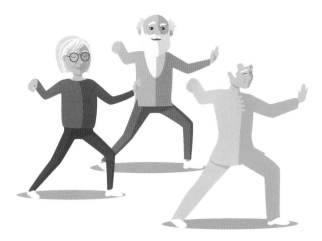

Tai chi involves maintaining different postures

Yoga focuses on meditation, slow movements, posture and breathing. It is similar to Tai chi, but rather than involving martial arts movements, yoga incorporates the holding of poses and mental concentration. Like Tai chi, the low-intensity nature of yoga means that it is suitable for older adults. A 2016 review of the literature found that yoga improved both balance and physical mobility in people aged 60 and over [4].

Long-term effects of exercise interventions on falls

Finnegan and team reviewed the long-term effects of exercise on fall prevention in older adults [5]. The researchers assessed the results of 24 studies, which included over 7,500 participants [5]. They found that exercise interventions can reduce both the rate and risk of falling, even after 12 months [5]. Finnegan and colleagues concluded that fall prevention exercise programmes resulted in a long-term

reduction of fall rates. This was maintained for up to two years after completion of the intervention [5]. This shows that even if there is a gap and failure to perform the exercise for a certain period, all is not lost, and one can restart the exercise when it becomes more convenient.

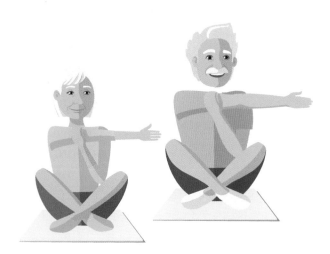

The effect of exercise in preventing falls can persist for a long period

References

1. Sherrington C, Fairhall NJ, Wallbank GK, et al. Exercise for preventing falls in older people living in the community. Cochrane Database Syst Rev. 2019;1(1):CD012424. Published 2019 Jan 31.
2. Robertson MC, Campbell AJ, Gardner MM, Devlin N. Preventing injuries in older people by preventing falls: a meta- analysis of individual-level data. J Am Geriatr Soc. 2002;50(5):905-911.
3. Wong AMK, Lan C. Tai Chi and balance control. Med Sport Sci. 2008;52:115-123.
4. Youkhana S, Dean CM, Wolff M, Sherrington C, Tiedemann A. Yoga-based exercise improves balance and mobility in people aged 60 and over: a

systematic review and meta-analysis. Age Ageing. 2016;45(1):21-29.

5. Finnegan S, Seers K, Bruce J. Long-term follow-up of exercise interventions aimed at preventing falls in older people living in the community: a systematic review and meta-analysis. Physiotherapy. 2019;105(2):187-199.

Metaphor 11 – How Often Should I Take My Pain Medication?

What is the story?
Prakash had a lovely garden. He heard on the news that it was going to be a scorching summer with very little rain for the next six months. Prakash realised that he needed to choose how he would care for his plants. His options were:

1. Never water his plants and just rely on the rain, if any.
2. Water the plants only when they were withering and dying.
3. Water the plants three times a day.
4. Water the plants twice a week.

So, what went wrong?
If Prakash opts for options one, two or three, it is likely that his plants won't survive. Options one and two provide "too little", and option three provides "too much". Option four provides the plants with adequate water for their needs.

How can we relate this story to our health?
If we experience pain, we need to take the recommended dosage of medication. Avoiding medications is not helpful. Similarly, delaying taking your pain medication until your pain is severe is also harmful, as shown by studies.

Moral of the story
Pain medication – Not too much, not too little, but just right.

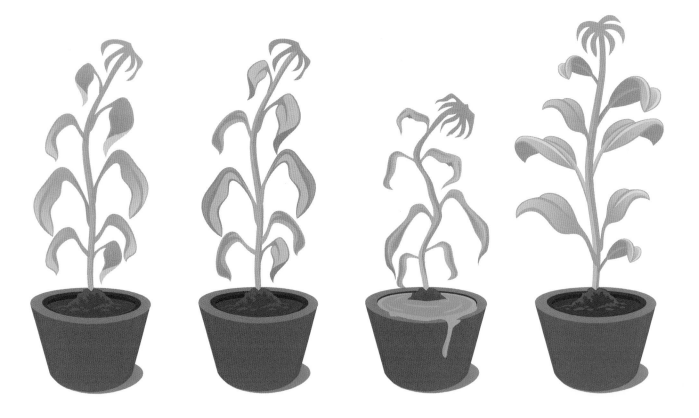

Reason 12 – Exercise Decreases Lower Back Pain

Lower back pain
Many people experience lower back pain (LBP). It is a common complaint in seniors and increases disability and creates functional limitations in later life. Most of the time, lower back pain resolves on its own within a few weeks. However, in some cases, the pain may become chronic. Chronic lower back pain is pain that lasts for more than three months. It affects nearly 20-25% of adults aged over 65 years and is the leading cause of disability worldwide.

Exercise and lower back pain
The study by Hicks and co-workers from the Tuscany region in Italy shows how group exercises can help with lower back pain. In their study, 392 adults between the ages of 50 and 88 participated in a physical activity programme for two days every week for a period of 12 months. More than 60% of the participants noticed that their back pain had improved during the 12-month period [1].

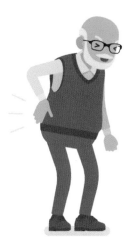

Back pain can frequently affect seniors

Exercise and Degenerative Spondylolisthesis (DS)
In the spine, vertebrae are arranged one over the other. Behind each vertebra is a ring of bone. All the rings, one over the other, form a canal through which the spinal cord and the nerves travel. In degenerative spondylolisthesis one of the lower lumbar vertebrae slips forwards. As the vertebra slips forward, the upper ring slips forward in relation to the lower ring. When one ring slips over the other, the space available for the nerves that pass through decreases. The edge of the ring traps the nerve as it slips forward, and this causes pain [2]. The narrowing of the space for the nerves is technically called stenosis.

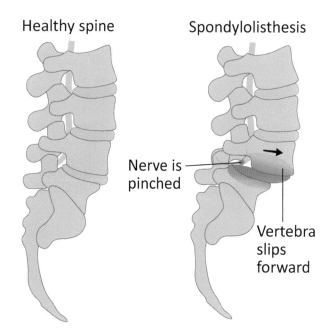

Healthy spine   Spondylolisthesis

Nerve is pinched

Vertebra slips forward

Degenerative spondylolisthesis, where one of the vertebrae slips forward, is the commonest cause of back pain and sciatica in seniors. Women are around five times more likely to develop this condition than men. The pressure on the nerve causes lower back pain and nerve pain down the legs (sciatica).

In the past few decades, surgery has become a popular intervention for degenerative spondylolisthesis. However, surgery is not absolutely necessary. A study published in 2017 investigated this by following 120 patients with moderate degenerative spondylolisthesis, with an average age of 68, for 3.3 years [3]. At the start and end of the study, participants were asked to report their leg and back pain on a 0-100 pain scale, where 0 is "no pain at all" and 100 is "as much pain as possible". In the 3.3 years, the leg pain of 32% of participants spontaneously improved without any surgery. Additionally, 36% of participants had spontaneous improvement of their back pain, again with no surgery [3]. The study concluded by supporting reluctance to surgery if the symptoms levels are tolerable for patients. The multi-centre SPORT trial [4] compared surgery and non-operative treatment for degenerative spondylolisthesis. 107 patients underwent surgery and 103 patients were treated none operatively and followed up for eight years. Pain and outcomes improved in both the groups over the period of eight years, but the improvement in the surgical group was better than the non-operative group. Oswestry Disability Index is measured on a scale of 0 to 100, where 0 indicates "not disabled" and 100 indicates "most severe disability". At the start of the study, the average disability of the patients was 42.4 [4]. Patients who underwent surgery decreased their disability by 18.1 points, while the non-surgical group decreased their disability by 7.9 points [4]. In summary, if non-surgical methods are not successful, then surgery could be considered.

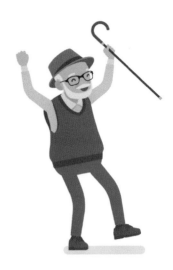

The leg pain in one-third of the patients improved spontaneously

There also exists some controversy on the type of exercises that need to be performed for degenerative spondylolisthesis. Some suggest flexion exercises (bending forwards and increasing the flexibility of the spine), whilst others suggest stabilisation exercises (strengthening rather than flexibility exercises). The study by Nava-Bringas and team investigated both these exercises. 92 patients over the age of 50, were randomly allocated to either lumbar stabilization exercises or flexion exercises [5]. Participants received six sessions of physical therapy (monthly appointments) and were instructed to execute the exercises at home each day during the six months of the study. Lower back and leg pain intensity were measured using the 0-100 pain scale described previously. These measures were taken before, during and after the intervention. After six months, both groups had reduced pain in the lower back by an average of 24.8 points on the 100-point scale. Both groups also reduced the pain felt in the legs by an average of 15.31 points. Additionally, disability was measured using the 0-100% Oswestry Disability Index (ODI). On this scale, a score closer to 100% means completely disabled and 0% means no disability. Following the exercises, participants in both groups reduced their disability scores by an average of 12.75% [5]. These results show that both lumbar stabilization and flexion exercises offer similar results with regards to controlling pain and decreasing disability in patients with degenerative spondylolisthesis.

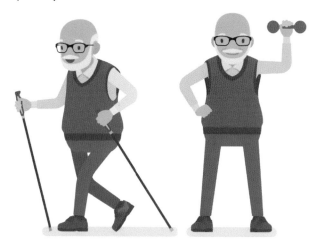

Aerobic and strengthening exercises can help with back and neck pain

References

1. Hicks GE, Benvenuti F, Fiaschi V, et al. Adherence to a community-based exercise program is a strong predictor of improved back pain status in older adults: an observational study. Clin J Pain. 2012;28(3):195-203.
2. Tenny S, Gillis CC. Spondylolisthesis. [Updated 2020 Jul 21]. In: StatPearls [Internet]. Treasure Island (FL): StatPearls Publishing; 2021 Jan-. Available from: https://www.ncbi.nlm.nih.gov/books/NBK430767/
3. Wessberg P, Frennered K. Central lumbar spinal stenosis: natural history of non-surgical patients. Eur Spine J. 2017;26(10):2536-2542.
4. Abdu WA, Sacks OA, Tosteson ANA, et al. Long-Term Results of Surgery Compared With Nonoperative Treatment for Lumbar Degenerative Spondylolisthesis in the Spine Patient Outcomes Research Trial (SPORT). Spine (Phila Pa 1976). 2018;43(23):1619-1630.
5. Nava-Bringas TI, Romero-Fierro LO, Trani-Chagoya YP, Macías-Hernández SI, García-Guerrero E, Hernández-López M, Coronado-Zarco R. Stabilization Exercises Versus Flexion Exercises in Degenerative Spondylolisthesis: A Randomized Controlled Trial [published online ahead of print, 2021 Apr 1]. Phys Ther. 2021;pzab108.

Metaphor 12 – How Do I Make My Back Strong?

What is the story?
Prabhu went camping with his family. They put up a tent and secured it with guy lines.

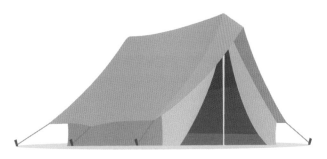

On the second morning, Prabhu noticed that the guy lines seemed to be slack, but since the tent pole was erect, he ignored the slack guy lines and did not tighten them.

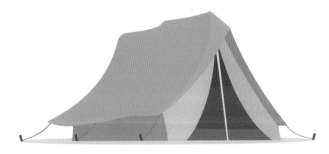

He went for a hike with his family. When they came back in the evening, the tent had completely collapsed.

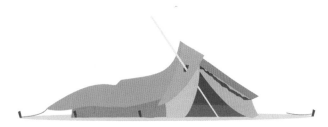

So, what went wrong?
The guy lines were slack in the morning. For the tent to remain standing, it needs both the pole and the guy lines. If the guy lines had been tightened, then the tent wouldn't have collapsed during the day. The guy lines need to be constantly tightened in order to support the tent.

How can we relate this story to our health?
We are only able to stand upright because of both the bones and the muscles which surround them. The bones by themselves will not be able to keep us upright. Similarly, the tent pole by itself cannot keep the tent erect. The guy lines are as important as the tent pole in keeping the tent erect. Similarly, our muscles are equally important as the bones in keeping us upright. Unfortunately, X-rays and MRI scans seem to focus on the bone and joints and ignore the muscle. Just as guy lines need to be constantly tightened, our muscles need regular exercise to keep them healthy and powerful, enabling them to provide the necessary support.

Moral of the story
For a strong back – regular exercise and maintenance help our muscles provide support.

Exercises for Neck Pain

Introduction

Patients with neck pain often complain that movement makes the pain worse. Despite this, most of the recommended exercises for neck pain use movement in an attempt to increase the range of motion and alleviate pain. This strategy actually increases the pain experienced and, as a result, patients with neck pain stop exercising. Not exercising makes the situation even worse.

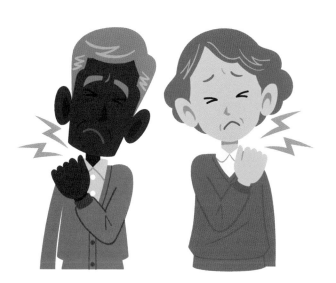

Thankfully, an alternative form of exercise is available. This different form of exercise is called isometric exercise. Isometric exercises strengthen muscles by engaging them in tension without movement. Patients are asked to resist the movement with their hands or elastic resistance bands to increase muscle strength. Once the strength is achieved, the range of movement will come naturally. Research shows that isometric and strengthening exercises of the neck and shoulder provide better relief than exercises that attempt to increase the range of movement [1, 2].

The above is like the chicken and the egg. In real life, we don't know which came first, the chicken or the egg. But in the case of exercises for neck pain, it is important to improve the strength before improving the range of motion. Attempting to increase the range of motion before increasing the strength will only result in more pain and noncompliance.

References

1. Gross A, Kay TM, Paquin JP, et al. Exercises for mechanical neck disorders. Cochrane Database Syst Rev. 2015;1:CD004250. Published 2015 Jan 28.
2. Liao CD, Tsauo JY, Huang SW, Ku JW, Hsiao DJ, Liou TH. Effects of elastic band exercise on lean mass and physical capacity in older women with sarcopenic obesity: A randomised controlled trial. Sci Rep. 2018;8(1):2317.

1 – Neck Extension

Intertwine the fingers of both hands and place your hands behind your head. Slowly push your head backwards into the palm of your hands whilst resisting this movement with your hands. In the beginning, only use a quarter of your maximum strength. You can slowly increase the force over the weeks. Hold for a count of ten. Then relax and rest your arms for a few seconds.
Repeat three times.

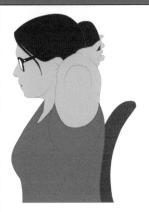

2 – Neck Flexion

Cup your hands together at the wrist and place them underneath your chin. Slowly push your head forward so that your chin is pushing into your cupped hands. Resist any movement of the head by using your hands. In the beginning, only use around a quarter of your maximum strength. You can slowly increase the force over the weeks. Hold for a count of ten. Then relax and rest your arms for a few seconds.
Repeat three times.

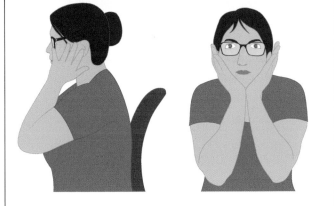

3 – Side Flexion

Place your right hand on the right side of your head above your ear. Attempt to tilt your head towards the right and resist that movement with your right hand. In the beginning, only use a quarter of your maximum strength. You can slowly increase the force over the weeks. Hold for a count of ten. Then relax and rest your arms for a few seconds.

Next, repeat the exercise on the left-hand side.

Performing this exercise once on the right side and once on the left side is one set. Perform three sets.

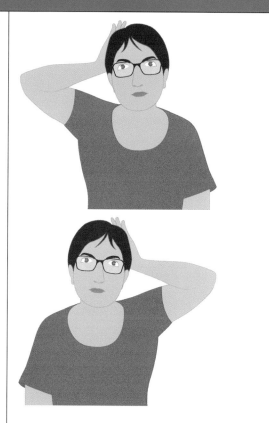

4 – Neck Rotation

Place your right palm on the side of your face. Attempt to turn your head to look over your right shoulder. Resist any movement of the head with your right hand. In the beginning, only use a quarter of your maximum strength. You can slowly increase the force over the weeks. Hold for a count of ten. Then relax and rest your arms for a few seconds.

Next, repeat the exercise on the left-hand side.

Performing this exercise once on the right side and once on the left side is one set. Perform three sets.

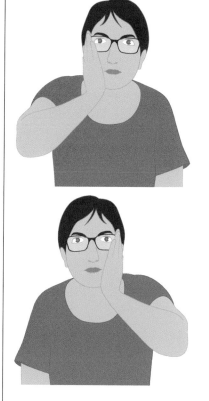

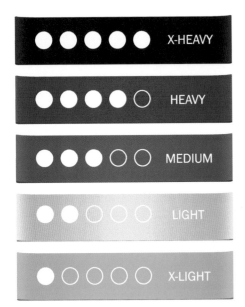

X-HEAVY

HEAVY

MEDIUM

LIGHT

X-LIGHT

A note about the exercise/resistance bands.

These can be purchased online or from any sports store. You need a straight band about 2 metres long to do the shoulder exercises. If you are very tall, you may need a longer band. The bands come in various degrees of thickness. The thicker the band is, the tougher they are to use. The colours may vary. The lighter colours typically are easier to use, whilst the darker colours are usually tougher, as shown in the diagram on the left. Err on the side of caution and use the lighter coloured bands to start with. The use of the band does come with its own added risk of injury. Therefore, please feel free to avoid these exercises. You will still be able to do a full-body exercise programme even without performing these particular exercises with the bands.

5 – Neck Extension With Resistance/Elastic Bands

Begin seated. Use a resistance/elastic resistance band and place it around the back of your head. If the band is slightly scrunched rather than completely flat, it will hold better. Hold your arms forwards with your elbows bent to a 90° angle and hold each limb of the resistance/elastic band with either hand. Hold the band without any slackness. It should stay put at the back of your head in this position but do not make any movements at this point. Then slowly pull the band forwards till your arms are straight.
Please ensure that the band does not snap up from the back of your head by tilting your head slightly backwards. It will take some time for you to find the right position. Please be careful to not cause yourself any harm. Resist the pull of the band by tensing the muscles at the back of your neck. Hold the position without moving for a count of ten. Then, relax and rest your arms for a few seconds.
Repeat three times.

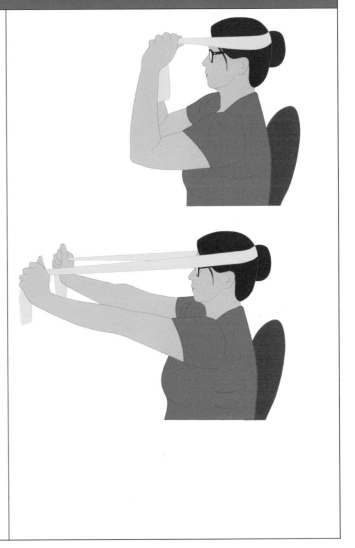

6 – Side Flexion With Resistance/Elastic Bands

Begin seated. Use a resistance/elastic band and place it around the left side of your head. If the band is slightly scrunched rather than completely flat, it will hold better. Lift your right arm sideways to the right with your elbows bent to a 90° angle and hold both limbs of the resistance/elastic band with your right hand. Hold the band without any slackness. It should stay put on the side of your head in this position but do not make any movements at this moment. Slowly pull the ends of the band to the right by straightening out your elbows. Please ensure that the band does not snap up from the side of your head or dig into your eyes. Take extreme care if you have had any surgery or issues with your eyes. It will take some time for you to find the correct position. Please be careful to not cause yourself any harm. Resist the pull of the band by tensing the muscles on the left side of your neck. Hold the position without moving for a count of ten. Then relax and rest your arms for a few seconds.

Next, repeat the exercise on the left-hand side.

Performing this exercise once on the right side and once on the left side is one set. Perform three sets.

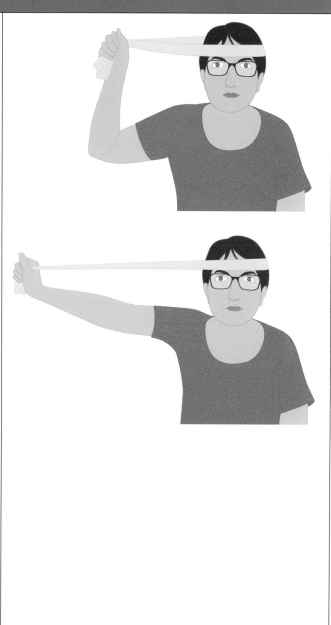

7 – Shoulder Thrust

Begin seated. Use a resistance/elastic band and place it around your back. Let the band come under your armpits and hold each limb of the band with either hand in front of your chest with your elbows bent.

There should not be any slack in the bands in this position. Now straighten out your elbows and stretch the band. Hold the position without moving for a count of ten. Then relax and rest your arms for a few seconds.

Repeat three times.

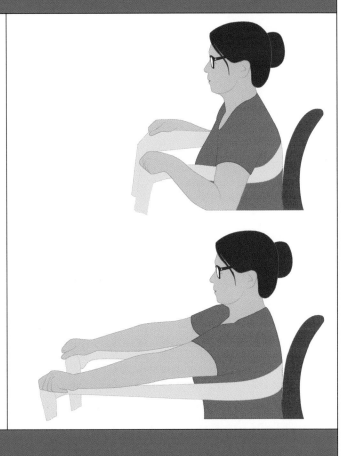

8 – Shoulder Lift

Begin seated. Use a resistance/elastic band and place it under both of your feet. Hold each limb of the band with each hand just beside your knees. There should not be any slack in the bands in this position. Lift your hands upwards whilst pulling upwards on the elastic resistance band. Go only as much as you can. Relax and return to the starting position.

Repeat ten times.

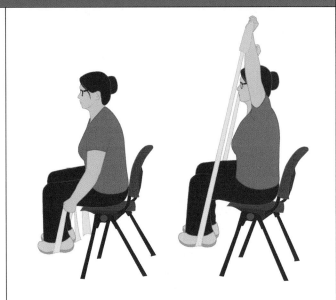

9 – Rowing With the Resistance Band

Begin seated. Use a resistance/elastic band and place it under both your feet. Hold each limb of the band with each hand just beside your knees. There should not be any slack in the band in this position. Pull your hands up towards your chest as if you are rowing. Relax and return to the starting position.
Repeat ten times.

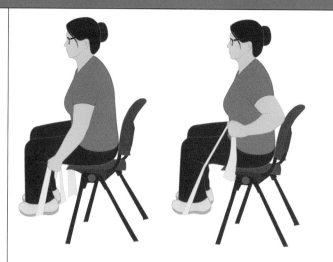

Exercises for Lower Back Pain

Introduction

Evidence suggests that a lack of muscle strength and coordination contributes to back pain. As a result, strengthening exercises have become a favoured prevention technique and treatment for back discomfort. Whilst there is an abundance of research into exercises for back pain, studies have struggled to find which exercise is best suited for lower back pain [1]. Even simple exercises such as running and Pilates can improve symptoms, but to perform these exercises when the pain is very intense may not be easy. For people with severe back pain, an alternative, less demanding form of exercise is required. This is where Motor Control Exercises (MCEs) may help. However, in order to understand why this is, we first need to understand the anatomy of the back. The back is mainly controlled by two groups of muscles – the multifidus and the erector spinae:

Multifidus (the stabilisers)

The multifidus is a muscle that runs up closest to the spine, attached at points to each vertebra. It provides stability and support to the spinal column. The fibres of this muscle are the first to become active to stabilise the spine even before we move.

Erector Spinae (the movers)

The erector spinae is a group of three large muscles that run outside the multifidus. The three muscles are the longissimus, the iliocostalis and the quadratus. Compared to the multifidus, the erector spinae muscles are large. Being large, they are able to exert great force and help us to bend and lift.

We need both the multifidus and the erector spinae to move. The multifidus stabilises the spine and the erector spinae move the spine. They have to come into play sequentially. First, the multifidus should contract and stabilise the spine. Then, the erector spinae should engage, which will then allow us to move the spine.

The problem

Unfortunately, following an injury or an episode of back pain, the multifidus muscle can become weak very quickly. On the other hand, the erector spinae do not become weak very easily. When the multifidus is weak, the erector spinae try to compensate. Unfortunately, the overcompensation by the erector spinae, without the multifidus first stabilising the vertebrae, creates abnormal stresses across the disc space and can lead to further discomfort and increases back spasms. This is why patients sometimes complain that any movement increases their back pain. They then do not do the exercise, which just compounds the

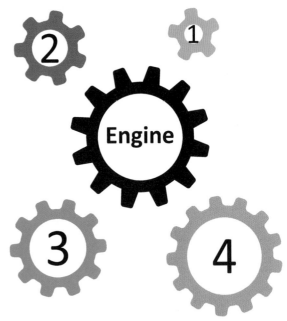

Schematic representation of a gearbox in a car engine

problem. Let me give a metaphor to help describe why this is: think of the muscles in our back as the gears in a car.

Let us imagine that the first gear is the multifidus muscle, as it is the first muscle that comes to play. The second, third and fourth gears are the different layers of the erector spinae muscles, as these come into play later. In order to move a car off, you need to engage the first gear and then change up through the gears in sequence, finally reaching fourth. However, imagine that the gearbox is faulty and that each time you attempt to engage the first gear, it automatically slips into the fourth gear. If this happens, the car will stall and will struggle to move off. This is the same as when our multifidus muscles are too weak to function properly. The erector spinae muscles will try to compensate by working harder. If the erector spinae act before the multifidus has stabilised the spine, it creates abnormal forces across the spine

and causes further pain. This is like the fourth gear engaging when we attempt to engage the first. In the car, the gearbox can be changed. In the back, we cannot change the muscles.

But the good news is that we can retrain the muscles in the back to return to the proper sequence. Pulling in the belly button (Abdominal drawing-in manoeuvre – ADIM) is a proven technique to retrain and re-strengthen the multifidus muscle.

MCEs

Motor-control exercises (MCEs) focus on re-training the deep local muscles of the multifidus so they become more active and stronger in movement [2]. Such exercises allow patients with back pain to regain the stability of their spine [3]. Motor-control exercises can also increase the size and density of the multifidus, decreasing recurrence and chronicity [4]. For example, repeatedly pulling in our belly button

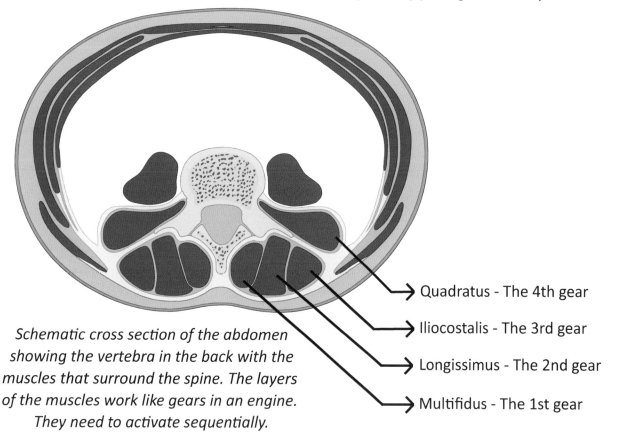

Quadratus - The 4th gear

Iliocostalis - The 3rd gear

Longissimus - The 2nd gear

Multifidus - The 1st gear

Schematic cross section of the abdomen showing the vertebra in the back with the muscles that surround the spine. The layers of the muscles work like gears in an engine. They need to activate sequentially.

towards our spine and pulling up the pelvic sling retrains the multifidus muscle, reducing the risk of injury or pain.

References

1. Rahman Shiri, David Coggon, Kobra Falah-Hassani. Exercise for the Prevention of Low Back Pain: Systematic Review and Meta-Analysis of Controlled Trials. Am J Epidemiol. 2018 May 1;187(5):1093-1101.
2. Rabin A, Shashua A, Pizem K, Dickstein R, Dar G. A clinical prediction rule to identify patients with low back pain who are likely to experience short-term success following lumbar stabilisation exercises: a randomised controlled validation study. J Orthop Sports Phys Ther. 2014;44(1):6-B13.
3. Bergmark A. Stability of the lumbar spine: A study in mechanical engineering. Acta Orthop Scand Suppl 1989; 230:1–54.
4. O'Sullivan PB, Phyty GD, Twomey LT, et al. Evaluation of specific stabilising exercise in the treatment of chronic low back pain with radiologic diagnosis of spondylolysis or spondylolisthesis. Spine 1997;22:2959–67.

Exercises for Lower Back Pain

1 – Engaging Your Core Whilst Sitting

Begin seated in an erect posture. Now draw in your belly button towards your spine and, at the same time, pull up the muscles in the floor of your pelvis (similar to the muscles you engage when trying not to go to the toilet). Hold this position for a count of ten. You can continue to breathe while holding the position. Release the position.

Repeat this ten times to complete one set. Perform three sets.

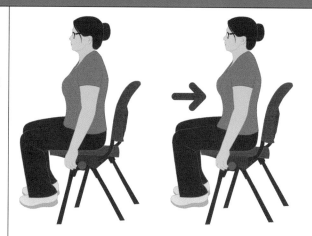

2 – Engaging Your Core Whilst Lying Down

Lie down on your back with your arms flat by your sides. You can do this exercise on the floor or on your bed. If on the bed, use a firm mattress. Bend your hips and knees and place your feet flat on the floor/mattress. Now draw in your belly button towards your spine and, at the same time, pull up the muscles in the floor of your pelvis (similar to the muscles you engage when trying not to go to the toilet).

Hold this position for a count of ten. You can continue to breathe while holding the position. Release the position.

Repeat this ten times to complete one set. Perform three sets.

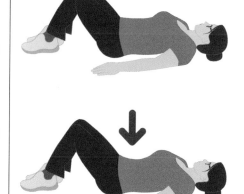

3 – Engaging Your Core Whilst on All Fours

Begin in the quadruped position (on your hands and knees). You can do this exercise on the floor or on your bed. If on the bed, use a firm mattress. Now draw in your belly button towards your spine and, at the same time, pull up the muscles in the floor of your pelvis (similar to the muscles you engage when trying not to go to the toilet). Hold this position for a count of ten. You can continue to breathe while holding the position. Release the position.
Repeat this ten times to complete one set. Perform three sets.

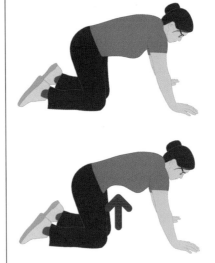

4 – Engaging Your Core Whilst Standing

Begin standing in an erect posture. Now draw in your belly button towards your spine and, at the same time, pull up the muscles in the floor of your pelvis (similar to the muscles you engage when trying not to go to the toilet). Hold this position for a count of ten. You can continue to breathe while holding the position. Release the position.
Repeat this ten times to complete one set. Perform three sets.

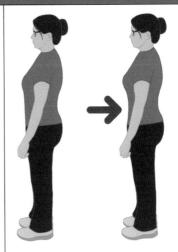

5 – Arm Lift Whilst on All Fours

Begin in the quadruped position (on your hands and knees). You can do this exercise on the floor or on your bed. If on the bed, use a firm mattress. Now draw in your belly button towards your spine and, at the same time, pull up the muscles in the floor of your pelvis. Then raise and stretch the right arm forwards. Hold this position for a count of ten. Relax and return the right arm to the original position.

Next, repeat the exercise on the left. Performing this exercise once on the right side and once on the left side is one set. Perform three sets.

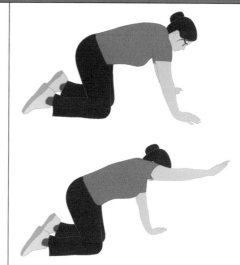

6 – Leg Lift Whilst on All Fours

Begin in the quadruped position (on your hands and knees). You can do this exercise on the floor or on your bed. If on the bed, use a firm mattress. Now draw in your belly button towards your spine and, at the same time, pull up the muscles in the floor of your pelvis. Then lift and stretch the right leg backwards so that leg is in line with the body and parallel to the floor. Hold this position for a count of ten. Relax and return the right leg to the original position.

Next, repeat the exercise on the left. Performing this exercise once on the right side and once on the left side is one set. Perform three sets.

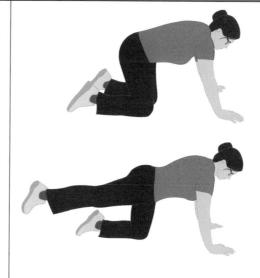

7 – Opposite Arm and Leg Lift Whilst on All Fours

Begin in the quadruped position (on your hands and knees). You can do this exercise on the floor or on your bed. If on the bed, use a firm mattress. Now draw in your belly button towards your spine and, at the same time, pull up the muscles in the floor of your pelvis. Then lift and stretch the left leg backwards so that leg is in line with the body and parallel to the floor. At the same time, lift the right arm forwards. Your right arm, your trunk and your left leg should all be in a straight line. Hold this position for a count of ten. Relax and return the leg and arm to the original position. Repeat the exercise for the opposite limbs.

Performing this exercise once with the right arm and left leg and once with the left arm and right leg is one set.

Perform three sets.

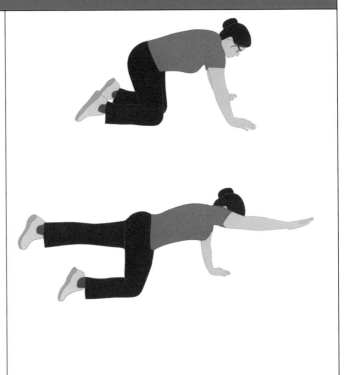

8 – Bridge or Supine Plank

Lie on your back with your arms by your side. You can do this exercise on the floor or on your bed. If on the bed, use a firm mattress. Bend your legs at the knee while keeping your feet flat on the floor. Now draw in your belly button towards your spine and, at the same time, pull up the muscles in the floor of your pelvis. Then push your hips up off the floor so that your trunk and thighs are in a straight line. Hold for a count of ten. Relax and lie back down on the floor/ bed. Repeat three times.

Advanced position: Instead of keeping your arms by your side, you can bend your elbow and keep your hands beside your ears. This makes it slightly more difficult than by keeping the arms by the side of the body.

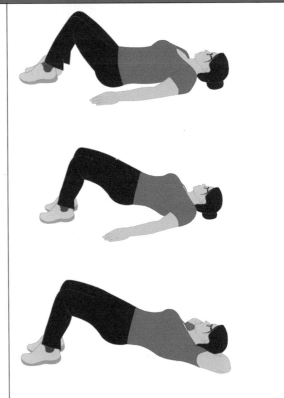

Otago Exercise Programme

Introduction

Otago Exercise Programme (OEP) is a home-based exercise programme that originated in New Zealand. Named after the region of the country where it was first developed, the programme was initially designed to improve balance and prevent falls in the elderly. The programme incorporates muscle strengthening and balance retraining exercises, with the aim to not only improve balance but also general fitness and well-being [1].

It was devised by Prof. Archibald John Campbell and Prof. Clare Robertson for the New Zealand Accident Compensation Corporation (ACC). This national corporation works with partners and other associations to help prevent injuries within the communities of New Zealand by funding research and rehabilitation [1].

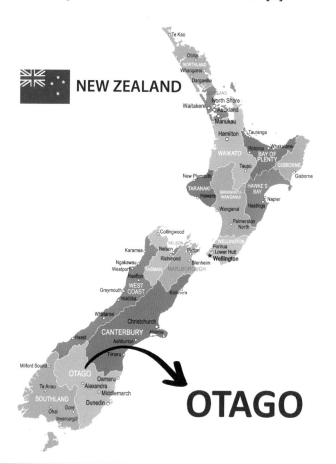

Most of the exercises within the programme can be carried out sitting down or holding onto the back of a chair. They focus mainly on the lower limbs and can be enhanced by using ankle weights. Ankle weights can be strapped to your ankles in order to increase the difficulty of the exercises. In the original study carried out by the developers, it was recommended that people over the age of 80 use ankle weights weighing 1-2 kg on each leg. Nevertheless, in these early trials, participants used up to 8 kg [1]. However, when we are attempting this programme, we must ensure that we do not 'boom and bust'. We must slowly progress from the lower weights up towards 8 kg through practice and hard work. Injuring ourselves by using weights that are too heavy too soon will only knock our confidence and hinder our progress.

Falls pose a huge threat to the health and welfare of older adults. It is estimated that, in the UK, 30% of adults over the age of 65 fall at least once every year. This statistic rises to 50% for people over 80 [2]. The physical and psychological effects of falls can be significant, and injuries sustained from falling are a leading cause of death [2]. The treatment and rehabilitation for such fall-related injuries place a significant financial burden on healthcare systems. For instance, approximately 5% of older people who fall sustain a fracture, with an estimated £2 billion spent annually on treatments from this fall injury alone. It is therefore imperative that fall prevention techniques are utilised as much as possible in order to reduce these statistics.

Studies support Otago Exercise Programme as an effective fall prevention technique.

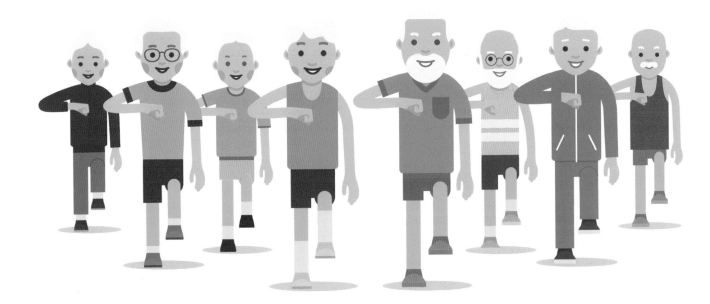

Research carried out by the inventors of the programme evaluated the effectiveness of the Otago Exercise Programme for adults aged between 65 and 97 years. The study found that the programme reduced falls and fall-related injuries by 35% [1]. A more recent study by Thomas and colleagues investigated the effect of the Otago Exercise Programme on the risk of death and fall rates in older adults (65+). The study found that the programme significantly reduced the risk of death whilst also considerably reducing fall rates [3].

Whilst fall prevention was the initial objective of the Otago Exercise Programme, it has now been heavily linked to improvements in the mobility and overall quality of life of those with arthritis. A study by Cederbom and colleagues required participants with arthritis to engage in a two-year Otago exercise programme. At the onset of the study, 86% of participants reported that they experienced moderate or extreme pain as a result of their arthritis. After the two years of participating in the Otago exercise programme, the proportion of participants experiencing such pain was reduced by 17% [4]. A further study by Mat and colleagues investigated the effects of Otago on seniors who were at an increased risk of falling and with knee osteoarthritis. They found that, by partaking in the Otago Exercise Programme, participants improved their pain and functionality. Participants' postural sway and directional control were also improved, reducing their risk of falling [5]. Otago has also been found to be cost effective when delivered to people aged 80 and above, with a return on investment of 127% [6].

In summary, not only is the Otago Exercise Programme a good fall prevention programme it also has benefits regarding musculoskeletal pain arising from arthritis - two birds with one stone. Furthermore, the programme is an excellent tool for reducing the following: fall associated injuries, the surgery that may be required to treat these injuries, the suffering and the resulting medical costs. The Otago Exercise Programme will not only benefit you but your society as a whole.

References

1. Robertson MC, Campbell AJ, Gardner MM, Devlin N. Preventing injuries in older people by preventing falls: a meta-analysis of individual-level data. *J Am Geriatr Soc*. 2002;50(5):905-911.

2. NICE. National Institute for Health and Care Excellence; London: 2013. Falls: assessment and prevention of falls in older people.

3. Thomas S, Mackintosh S, Halbert J. Does the 'Otago exercise programme' reduce mortality and falls in older adults?: a systematic review and meta-analysis. *Age Ageing*. 2010;39(6):681-687.

4. Cederbom S, Arkkukangas M. Impact of the fall prevention Otago Exercise Programme on pain among community-dwelling older adults: a short- and long-term follow-up study. *Clin Interv Aging*. 2019;14:721-726.

5. Mat S, Ng CT, Tan PJ, et al. Effect of Modified Otago Exercises on Postural Balance, Fear of Falling, and Fall Risk in Older Fallers With Knee Osteoarthritis and Impaired Gait and Balance: A Secondary Analysis. *PM R*. 2018;10(3):254-262.

6. Carande-Kulis V, Stevens J.A, Florence C.S, Beattie B.L, Arias I.J. A cost-benefit analysis of three older adult fall prevention interventions. Safety Res. 2015 Feb;52:65-70.

1 – Sitting and Marching - Warm Up

Begin seated. Now, start marching using your arms and legs. Sitting and marching is slightly more difficult than standing and marching, but it will get easier with practice. The difficulty is in coordinating the movement of your arms and legs. Make sure to lift your right leg whilst lifting your left arm and vice versa. Make sure you don't lapse into lifting both your right arm and right leg (or the left arm and left leg) at the same time. Continue marching for a minute or two.

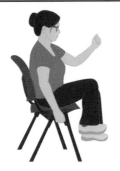

2 – Standing From Seated Position - Hip Walk and Stand

It is easier to stand up from a seated position if your bottom is closer to the front of the seat and the knees are slightly bent and feet slightly tucked inwards. To get to this position, you need to 'hip walk'. Hip walking involves moving the right side of your bottom slightly forward, followed by the left side. Do this a few times until you are sitting towards the front of your seat. Make sure that you do not move yourself too far forward, as you may risk falling off your chair. Once you have reached the front of the seat, bend your knees a little and tuck your feet in slightly – this helps you to stand. Gain support by putting your hands on your thighs or on the arms of the chair. Push down onto your thighs or the arms of your chair with your hands and stand up. Once you have practised this, you will not need the help of your hands.

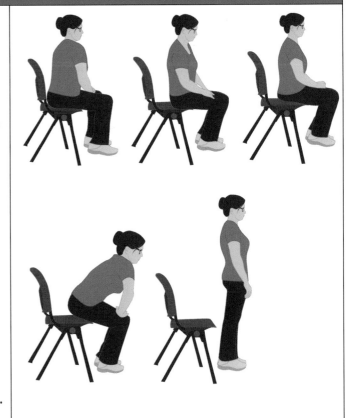

3 – Head Turns

Begin standing behind your chair. If you prefer, you can hold onto the backrest for support.

Turn your head slowly to the right so that you are looking over your right shoulder. Go only as far as you can and then return to facing forwards. Now turn your head to the left to look over your left shoulder. Make sure to take a momentary pause when you reach the centre (facing forwards) instead of just making a continuous movement from left to right or right to left.

Repeat the full sequence five times.

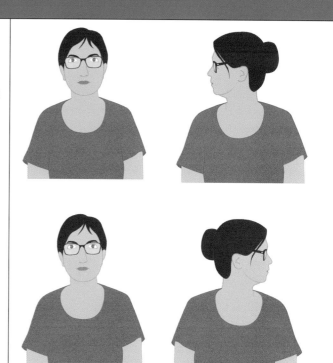

4 – Neck Glides

Begin standing. Hold your hand two inches away from your face at the height of your chin. Keeping your hand in the same place, move your head forward to touch your outheld hand with your lips. Then relax your neck and return your head back to its normal position.

Repeat five times.

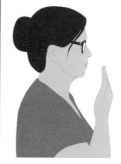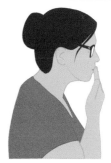

5 – Trunk Turns

Begin standing. Place both your arms across your chest in an 'X' formation so that each hand is placed on the opposite shoulder. Now rotate your trunk and turn your chest to the right whilst making sure you do not rotate your hips or neck. Only rotate your trunk. Return to the start position and then turn to the left. Once again, return to the start position.

Repeat five times.

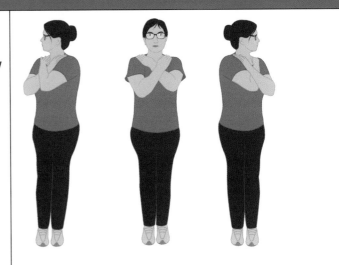

6 – Back Extension

Begin standing behind a chair so that you can hold on to the back of the chair if you need support. Place both your hands on the back of your hips. Look directly forward and focus on one point at eye level in front of you. Now gently push your hips forward and arch your back into a gentle curve. Return to the erect posture. Ensure that you keep looking forward throughout and do not look upwards when pushing your hips forward.

Repeat five times.

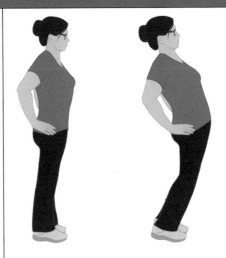

7 – Ankle Movements

Begin seated. Keep your feet flat on the floor, positioned slightly away from you, with a slight bend in your knees. Now pull up the front of both of your feet so that your toes are off the floor and only your heels remain grounded.
Then, relax and return your feet flat on the floor.
Repeat five times.

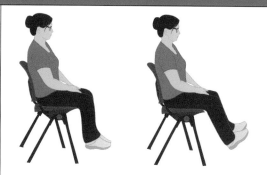

Please put on your ankle weights for the next 3 exercises

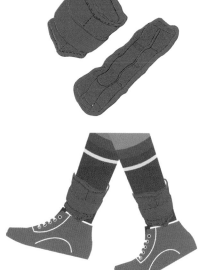

You can buy ankle weights from any sports store or online. They come in various sizes but it's best to start at a low weight of around 1kg on each leg and then work your way up as you develop more strength. Before wearing your ankle weights, make sure you are wearing full length trousers that cover your ankles or alternatively thick socks that come up to your shins - this is to protect your skin when you put the weights on. It's best to put them on in a seated position, before standing up and assessing for comfort. Make sure that they are fitted but not too tight - this can be adjusted on the strap itself. Ensure to only wear them when recommended within the exercise guide, and remove them when not needed. If you have ulcers, surgical scars or any other injury around your ankles or feet we advise that you do not wear the ankle weights. You will still be able to complete most of the exercise programme even if you do not use the weights.

8 – Front Knee Strengthener

Begin seated with your ankle weights attached and both knees bent. Now, slowly straighten your right knee by lifting your lower leg. Once your right leg is fully straightened, slowly bend your right knee to return to the starting position.
Repeat five times for each leg.

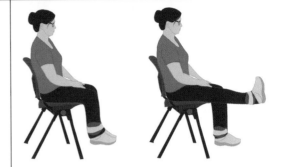

9 – Back Knee Strengthener

Begin standing with your ankle weights strapped on. If you want, you can hold onto the backrest of a chair for support. Whilst standing, bend your right leg backwards at the knee and bring your foot up to a horizontal position. Once your lower leg is at a right angle with your thigh, lower your foot slowly to the floor. It is important that you are lifting the foot backwards by only bending at the knee.
Ensure that whilst doing this movement you don't move your thigh/knee forward.
Repeat five times for each leg.

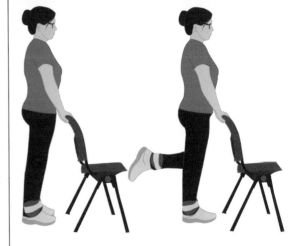

10 – Side Hip Strengthener

Begin standing with your ankle weights strapped on. If you prefer, you can hold onto the backrest of a chair for support. Now, lift your entire left leg out to the left side. Ensure that your leg is straight and your toes are pointing forwards. You should make sure to use your gluteal muscles, which are on the side of your hip. The tendency is to turn your toes in the same direction that you are moving your leg, but unfortunately, this then engages a different muscle. To always use the gluteus medius, you should keep your toes pointing forwards at all times. Move your foot back down to the original starting position. Repeat five times for each leg.

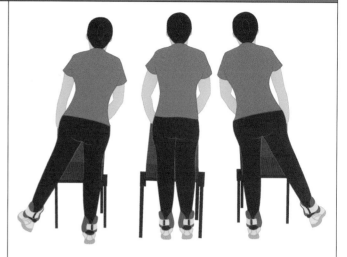

You can now remove your ankle weights

11 – Heel Raises – Tiptoeing

Begin standing behind the back of a chair. If you wish, you can hold onto the backrest for support. Stand straight with your feet slightly apart. Now slowly raise both your heels off the ground until you are on your tiptoes. Then slowly lower yourself down.
Repeat five times.

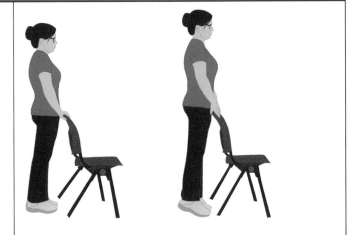

12 – Toe Raises

Begin standing behind the back of a chair. If you prefer, you can hold onto the backrest for support. Stand straight with your feet slightly apart. Now raise your toes of both feet slowly off the ground until you are resting on your heels only. Then, slowly lower your toes back down to the floor.
Repeat five times.

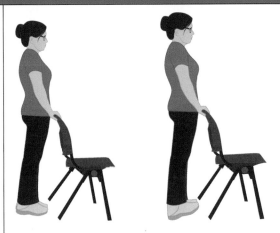

13 – Knee Bends – Supported

Begin standing in front of a chair. If you want more support, place another chair in front of you. You can hold onto the backrest of the chair if needed. Stand straight with your feet slightly apart and pointing forwards. Start by bending at both the knees and hips, pushing your buttocks backwards as if you were about to sit down. Try to keep your knees directly above your feet. Stop when you have reached halfway between the standing and sitting position and then return to the starting position. Ensure that your buttocks do not hit the seat.

Repeat five times. If you initially need the supporting chair in front, practice will enable you to eventually do this exercise without it (advanced version).

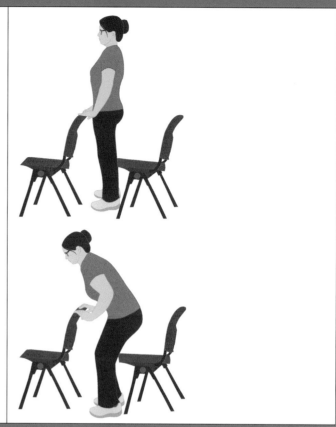

14 – Sit to Stand – Supported

Using the "hip walk" manoeuvre described in Exercise 2, move forward to the front of your seat. Bend your knees and tuck your feet slightly. Gain support by pushing down onto your legs/sides of the chair with your hands and stand up. Once you are standing upright, slowly sit down again, placing your hands on your knees or the sides of the chair for support.

Repeat five times. In the future, you may be able to do this exercise without using your hands for support (advanced version).

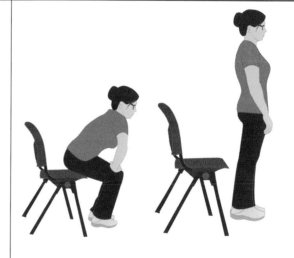

15 – Heel Toe Stand (Tandem)

Begin standing upright beside the back of a chair with your side adjacent to the backrest. If you prefer, you can hold onto the backrest for support. Now, place the left foot directly in front of the right foot. The toes of the right foot will be touching the heel of the left. Spread your weight evenly between both feet. Please do not lock your knees straight. Stand straight and hold this position for a count of ten. Then, move your left foot back to the original position. Repeat with the right foot being in front. You may eventually be able to do this exercise without the support of the chair (advanced version).

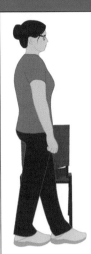

16 – Heel Toe Walking

Begin standing adjacent to the back of a row of chairs/a table. If needed, hold onto the backrest/table for support. Walk in tandem, placing one foot in front of the other, so the heel and toes touch to form a straight line. Keep your posture as tall and straight as possible. Walk ten steps. If you do not have room to walk ten steps, stop when you reach the end of the length of the table or chairs. Turn around and walk ten steps in the same manner to return to the starting position. With practice, you may be able to do this exercise without the support of the chair/table (advanced version).

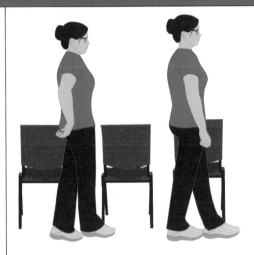

17 – Single Leg Stand

Begin standing beside the back of a chair with your side adjacent to the backrest. Now raise the right foot off the ground by bending slightly at the hip and knee. Keep your left leg straight, but do not lock the knee. Hold for a count of ten and then lower your right foot to the floor. Repeat with the opposite leg. If you initially need the support of the chair, practice may eventually allow you to do this unsupported (advanced version).

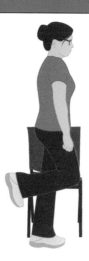

18 – Sideways Walking

Begin standing upright behind a row of chairs/a table. Hold onto the backrest/table for support. Step sideways to the right with your right foot. Then follow with the other foot so that both the feet end up together. Walk ten steps in this way. If you do not have room to walk ten steps, stop when you reach the end of the length of the table or chairs. Then step sideways in the opposite direction leading with your other foot to return to the starting position to finish. You may eventually be able to do this exercise without the need of the supporting chairs/table (advanced version).

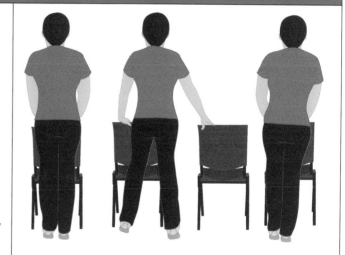

19 – Toe Walking

Begin standing adjacent to the back of a row of chairs/a table. Hold onto the backrest/table for support.

Tiptoe and walk forward on your toes. Walk ten steps. If you do not have room to walk ten steps, stop when you reach the end of the length of the table or chairs. Turn around and, using the back of the chairs as support, walk a further ten steps to return to the start position to finish. Ensure to keep your heels off the floor while you do this exercise. With practice, you may eventually be able to do this exercise without the rows of chairs/tables for support (advanced version).

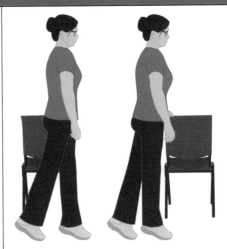

20 – Heel Walking

Begin standing behind and beside a row of chairs/a table. Hold onto the backrest/table for support. Lift the toes and front of the feet off the floor. Using the back of the chairs/table as support, walk forward on your heels.

Walk ten steps. If you do not have room to walk ten steps, stop when you reach the end of the length of the table or chairs. Turn around and, using the back of the chairs/table as support, walk a further ten steps to return to the starting position to finish. Ensure to keep your toes and the front of your feet off the floor while you do this exercise. By practising, you may be able to do this exercise without the chairs/table for support (advanced version).

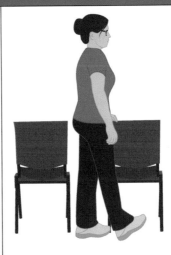

21 – Walking Backwards – Supported

Begin standing adjacent to the back of a row of chairs/a table. Hold onto the backrest/table for support. Walk backwards for ten steps. If you do not have room to walk ten steps, stop when you reach the end of the length of the table or chairs. Turn around and then walk backwards ten steps to return to the starting position to finish. After practising this exercise, you may be able to do it without the use of the chair/table for support (advanced version).

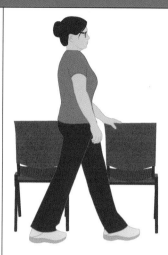

22 – Heel-to-Toe Walking Backwards – Supported

Begin standing adjacent to the back of a row of chairs/a table. Hold onto the backrest/table for support. Walk backwards for ten steps in tandem, i.e. the toe touching the heel of the other foot. If you do not have room to walk ten steps, stop when you reach the end of the length of the table or chairs. Then, turn around and walk backwards in tandem for ten steps to return to the starting position to finish. You may eventually be able to do this exercise without the need for the supporting chairs/table (advanced version).

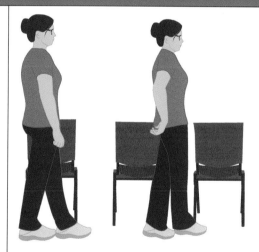

23 – Walk and Turn

Arrange two chairs side-by-side, leaving a gap which you can safely walk through. Stand next to one of the chairs and walk around both the chairs in a figure of eight. Repeat this process twice.

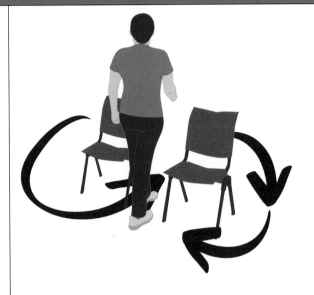

24 – Stair Walking

Hold onto the bannister for support and climb up a flight of stairs. Turn around and, holding onto the bannister, climb back down the flight of stairs. Repeat this process twice.

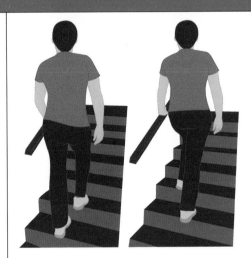

25 – Calf Stretch

Using the "hip walk" manoeuvre shown in Exercise 2, move forward to the front of your seat. Keep your left knee bent with your left foot on the floor and straighten your right leg at the knee. Now pull your toes and the front of your right foot towards you. Pull until you feel the stretch in the back of your right calf. Hold for a count of ten and then relax your right foot. Repeat with the other leg.

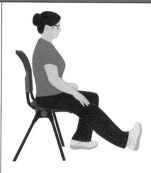

26 – Stretching the Back of the Thigh

Using the "hip walk" manoeuvre shown in Exercise 2, move forward to the front of your seat. Keep your left knee bent with your left foot on the floor and straighten your right leg at the knee. Place both your hands on your right thigh. Slowly slide your hands down the front of your thigh and leg towards your foot. Ensure you keep your trunk as straight as possible. Push forward till you feel the stretch in the back of your thigh. Hold for a count of ten and then return to the starting position. Repeat with the other leg.

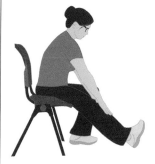

27 – Knee Bends – No Support (Advanced Version of 13)

Begin standing in front of a chair. Stand straight with your feet slightly apart and pointing forwards. Start by bending at both the knees and hips, pushing your buttocks backwards as if you were about to sit down. Try to keep your knees directly above your feet. Stop when you have reached halfway between the standing and sitting position and then return to the starting position.
Repeat five times.

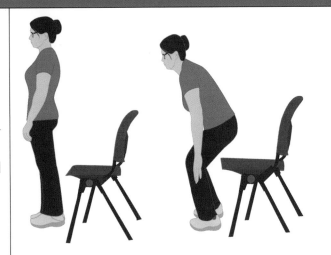

28 – Sit to Stand – No Support (Advanced Version of 14)

Using the "hip walk" manoeuvre shown in Exercise 2, move forward to the front of your seat. Bend your knees and tuck your feet slightly. Thrust down with your legs and stand up. Once you have stood upright, slowly sit down again. Repeat five times.

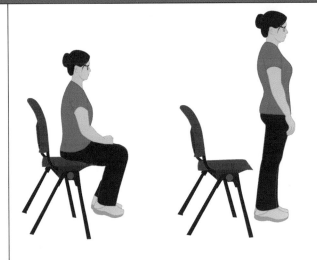

29 – Heel Toe Stand (Tandem) – No Support (Advanced Version of 15)

Begin standing upright. Now place your left foot directly in front of your right foot. The toes of your right foot should be touching the heel of your left foot. Spread your weight evenly between both your legs. Do not lock your knees straight. Stand straight and hold this position for a count of ten. Then, move your left foot back to the original position. Repeat with your right foot being in front.

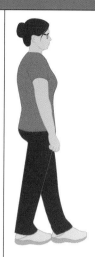

30 – Heel Toe Walking – No Support (Advanced Version of 16)

Begin standing upright. Walk ten steps forwards in tandem, placing one foot in front of the other. The heel of one foot should touch the toe of the other to form a straight line. Turn around and walk ten steps, in the same manner, to return to the starting position to finish.

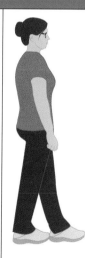

31 – Single Leg Stand – No Support (Advanced Version of 17)

Begin standing upright. Now raise your left foot off the ground. Keep your right leg straight, but do not lock the knee. Hold for a count of ten and then lower your left foot to the floor. Repeat the same with the opposite leg.

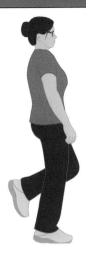

32 – Sideways Walking – No Support (Advanced Version of 18)

Begin standing upright. Step sideways to the right with your right foot. Then, follow with the left foot so that both of your feet are together. Using these steps, move ten steps to the right. Then, take ten steps in the opposite direction leading with the left foot, to return to the starting position to finish.

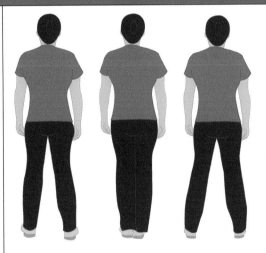

33 – Toe Walking – No Support (Advanced Version of 19)

Begin standing upright. Tiptoe and walk forward on your toes for ten steps. Turn around and walk a further ten steps to return to the start position to finish. Ensure you keep your heels off the floor while doing this exercise.

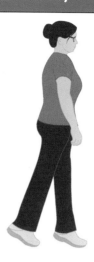

34 – Heel Walking – No Support (Advanced Version of 20)

Begin standing upright. Lift your toes and the front of your foot off the floor. Walk forward on your heels for ten steps. Turn around and walk a further ten steps to return to the starting position to finish. Keep your toes and the front of your feet off the floor while doing this exercise.

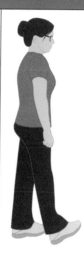

35 – Walking Backwards – No Support (Advanced Version of 21)

Begin standing upright. Step backwards for ten steps. Turn around and then walk backwards ten steps to return to the starting position to finish.

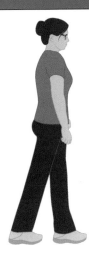

36 – Heel-to-Toe Walking Backwards – No Support (Advanced Version of 22)

Begin standing upright. Walk backwards for ten steps in tandem, i.e., the toe touching the heel of the opposite foot. Then turn around and walk backwards in tandem for ten steps to return to the starting position to finish.

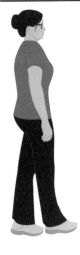

Exercise Diary

Exercise Diary Name .... Date of starting programme..........................

Week 1	Monday	Tuesday	Wed	Thursday	Friday	Saturday	Sunday
Date							
Exercise (Yes / No)							
Any falls?							

Week 2	Monday	Tuesday	Wed	Thursday	Friday	Saturday	Sunday
Date							
Exercise (Yes / No)							
Any falls?							

Week 3	Monday	Tuesday	Wed	Thursday	Friday	Saturday	Sunday
Date							
Exercise (Yes / No)							
Any falls?							

Week 4	Monday	Tuesday	Wed	Thursday	Friday	Saturday	Sunday
Date							
Exercise (Yes / No)							
Any falls?							

Week 5	Monday	Tuesday	Wed	Thursday	Friday	Saturday	Sunday
Date							
Exercise (Yes / No)							
Any falls?							

Week 6	Monday	Tuesday	Wed	Thursday	Friday	Saturday	Sunday
Date							
Exercise (Yes / No)							
Any falls?							

Exercise Diary

Name .... Date of starting programme.........................

Week 7	Monday	Tuesday	Wed	Thursday	Friday	Saturday	Sunday
Date							
Exercise (Yes / No)							
Any falls?							

Week 8	Monday	Tuesday	Wed	Thursday	Friday	Saturday	Sunday
Date							
Exercise (Yes / No)							
Any falls?							

Week 9	Monday	Tuesday	Wed	Thursday	Friday	Saturday	Sunday
Date							
Exercise (Yes / No)							
Any falls?							

Week 10	Monday	Tuesday	Wed	Thursday	Friday	Saturday	Sunday
Date							
Exercise (Yes / No)							
Any falls?							

Week 11	Monday	Tuesday	Wed	Thursday	Friday	Saturday	Sunday
Date							
Exercise (Yes / No)							
Any falls?							

Week 12	Monday	Tuesday	Wed	Thursday	Friday	Saturday	Sunday
Date							
Exercise (Yes / No)							
Any falls?							

Printed in Great Britain
by Amazon

85830458R00056